Say No to ASTHMA

Cure asthma through change in diet and lifestyle

Jonathan M Berkowitz, MD

Vitasta

Vitasta Publishing Pvt. Ltd.
New Delhi

Times Group Books

The information contained in this book is based upon the research and personal and professional experiences of the author. It is not intended as a substitute for consulting with your physician or other healthcare provider. Any attempt to diagnose and treat an illness should be done under the direction of a healthcare professional. The publisher does not advocate the use of any particular healthcare protocol but believes the information in this book should be available to the public.

The publisher and author are not responsible for any adverse effects or consequences resulting from the use of the suggestions, preparations, or procedures discussed in this book. Should the reader have any questions concerning the appropriateness of any procedures or preparation mentioned, the author and the publisher strongly suggest consulting a professional healthcare advisor.

Marketed and Distributed exclusively in India & Sub-Continent by:

Times Group Books

Times Group Books
(A division of Bennett, Coleman and Company Limited)
Times Annexe, Express Building
9-10 Bahadur Shah Zafar Marg, New Delhi- 110 002

Published by:

Vitasta

Vitasta Publishing Pvt. Ltd.
2/15, Ansari Road, Daryaganj, New Delhi-110 002

ISBN 978-93-80828-07-7

First Published by Basic Health Publications, Inc, US, as
Asthma: Relax You're not Going to Die

Editor: John Anderson

Cover Design and Layout by Vitasta Publishing Pvt. Ltd.
Printed by Vits Press, New Delhi (India)

Contents

For Cecilia, My Wife

For Daniel, My Son

My Light, My Joy

Introduction

My Story and a Few Basic Lessons

I HAVE TROUBLE SAYING THIS, but asthma saved my life. Before I accepted the fact that I had asthma, I was fooling myself that the consequences of an amazingly unhealthy lifestyle would never catch up with me. By age twenty-three, I had chalked up a decade of smoking cigarettes, religiously avoided exercise, and subsisted on a diet that would give the American Heart Association a coronary. In other words, to any intelligent observer, it was obvious that I was looking forward to a heart attack by age forty.

Another confession: I never expected to be alive today. At twenty-three, I got sick, very sick. According to the doctors, I had severe asthma, and I rapidly became steroid dependent. During my most intense treatment, I was on seven different medications, including steroids. I gained fifty pounds, the weight gain being so rapid that I got stretch marks on my stomach, underarms, and thighs. I knew the steroids were destroying my body, and I fully expected to be wheelchair-bound or dead by age thirty-five. I called steroids the "die now or die later plan." My only hope was that my asthma would simply go away or a medical "miracle" would cure me.

In retrospect, I probably had asthma from childhood. I had trouble playing sports, always running out of breath before the other children. My real problems, however, began when I started smoking at age thirteen. Before then, I would catch the usual winter colds, which would quickly resolve after several days. After I started smoking, my colds became severe, evolving into weeks of bronchitis. Yet, my addiction to nicotine was so strong that I kept smoking. At fifteen, after one particularly nasty cold, my doctor told me I had asthma—"Stop smoking and it will go away," he said. I just laughed at him.

Such is the bravado of youth. Well, everything caught up with me during my last year of college. On Easter Sunday, my girlfriend and I bought a rabbit as a house pet. It may surprise some of you to learn that rabbits can be potty trained, and that is where my troubles went from bad to worse. With the rabbit came a litter box with aromatic, shaved cedar chips. Literally hours after making "Bumpers the Bunny" a home, I began to get this weird sensation in my chest, a strange heaviness that took my breath away. As was my usual modus operandi, I ignored these symptoms. Nothing could be wrong with me—I was a twenty-three-year-old indestructible male living the American Dream.

At first these symptoms appeared only at home; however, over a period of weeks my symptoms became nearly constant. After some questionable reasoning, I came to the conclusion that my complaints could be blamed on allergies, it being peak allergy season in Connecticut, where I was living at the time. Yet, my symptoms were becoming more severe and, even worse, they interfered with my smoking. I wasn't about to stand for that! After a month of misery, I found myself in an allergist's office. After listening to my story and my lungs, it was quickly apparent to him that I had asthma.

Hindsight and knowledge have made my condition crystal clear but no less painful. As a physician, when I see a person who has his or her asthma "destabilized" or has "new-onset" asthma, my first questions are always: Is there anything new in your life? Have you been sick with a cold? Do you have a new pet or a new significant other? Many times, questions like these can uncover the source of the problem and, as you will learn in Chapter 6, removing the source of irritation is the best defense against asthma.

Unfortunately, my allergist didn't ask these fundamental questions and, to this day, I remain surprised and disappointed that he didn't shake me and say, "Dump the bunny, Berkowitz, and you'll feel better." Instead, after the usual admonishment about smoking, I left his office with two inhalers and a prescription for prednisone.

LESSON ONE: DOCTORS ARE ONLY HUMAN

Despite all its shortcomings, despite all its failures, conventional Western medicine is a wonderful thing. There is no question that without doctors and drugs, many people who are walking the Earth today would not be here. Asthma is a case in point. Despite the fact that there are many asthmatics who are overmedicated, inappropriately medicated, or made even worse by medication, there are millions of asthmatics alive and well today who can thank Western medicine for their health. Doctors are usually smart people who want to do good, but are human just like you and me. As the scars on my body will attest, I know firsthand that doctors can make mistakes. Pointing fingers, however, is not what this book is about. What you can expect to learn is how to change your life and rid yourself of asthma. In the process of exorcising asthma from your body, I hope you will become medication-free or, at the very least, significantly reduce the amount of medication you use. Even more important, I hope that the lessons learned in this book will enable you to lead a more healthy and active life.

LESSON TWO: AN OUNCE OF PREVENTION IS WORTH A POUND OF CURE

One of modern medicine's shortcomings is its reliance on technology and drugs. Too many doctors wait for disease to manifest before acting, rather than preventing disease in the first place. My doctor's fundamental mistake was that he relied too heavily on medicine to take care of the problem, instead of demanding that I make some tough life decisions. He saw his role as diagnosing the patient's condition, prescribing pills A, B, and C, and sending the patient home. The use of medicine in healthcare, at least from my perspective, is not that simple. These are exciting times for modern medicine because there is a growing consensus among the new generation of doctors that healthcare is a partnership between doctor and patient. That, yes, technology and medications play a vital role, but the real benefit rests with prevention. If we can prevent a condition from developing, we won't have to worry about treating it in the future.

Allow me to get off the asthma track for a moment to illustrate the importance of prevention. Heart disease is America's number one killer of men and women. In my practice, I see far too many people with heart problems. Here's the real tragedy: For the overwhelming majority of people, heart disease is preventable—no one should die of a heart attack. What causes heart attacks? Most are caused by tobacco, high cholesterol, and lack of exercise. In other words, most heart attacks are caused by bad living. There are three basic choices we all make that influence our chances of having a heart attack:

1. To exercise or not to exercise
2. To smoke or not to smoke

3. To eat a healthy or an unhealthy diet

Make the right choices and, chances are, you'll live to a ripe old age. Even better news: If you live a healthy life, the vast majority of diseases, including asthma, can be prevented or at least better controlled. Heart attacks are really a sign of failure—failure of the patient to live healthy and failure of the healthcare system to use its wisdom to prevent a disaster.

This brings me back to my encounter with the allergist, who would become first in a long line of doctors. As a patient, I failed because I knew smoking was bad for my health yet I continued to smoke. My doctor failed because he didn't take the time to see my symptoms in the context of my overall life situation and elected to take the easy road by giving me a couple of inhalers and a handful of steroids and sending me on my way. Moral of the story: Medicine is a two-way street. Always think about what you can do to help yourself, and always ask your doctor what you can do to solve the problem.

So there I was, pills and inhalers in hand, confident that they would save me. Like so many people, I put all my faith in the medical profession. Here's the amazing part: I had just been diagnosed with a potentially chronic and deadly condition and it didn't bother me. I figured, if I followed my doctor's advice, everything would be OK. But after three weeks, my symptoms only got worse and Bumpers the Bunny remained cuter than ever. Then I did something smart—I went to another doctor, a pulmonary specialist.

This doctor did the usual history and physical exam, and some performed breathing. While this doctor wasn't thrilled that I was placed on steroids from the start, steroids usually being the drugs of last resort, he was concerned that I wasn't getting better. He suggested that, along with quitting smoking, I should start to taper off the steroids. In the meantime, he would put me on several new medicines to help me "get over the steroids." Once again, the doctor asked no questions about my home or gave even the slightest hint that dumping Bumpers the Bunny might help.

From this seemingly innocent beginning, a vicious cycle began: several years of going on and off steroids and trying medication after medication. By the time I got fed up with this doctor, I was on seven different medications, including steroids. While my asthma mercifully did not get worse, it did not get better either. And emotionally, I was a wreck. One week I would be off the steroids only to catch a cold the next week and have to go right back on them. Not only did this merry-go-round of pill popping play havoc with my emotions, the steroids made me hyperactive, irritable, and emotionally labile. I would cry every time I had to start back on the steroids, wondering if my body would ever allow me to stop.

My asthma outlasted my girlfriend who got the rabbit while I got to keep my asthma. Guess what I did? Being so heartbroken, I went out and bought myself a new rabbit—amazing the stupid things people do! As it turns out, my new rabbit didn't last long. I decided to go to medical school and promptly moved to New York City to do preparatory studies at Columbia University. Since New York City apartments and bunnies don't mix, my rabbit found himself adopted by a loving family. One thing I didn't get rid of was my doctor and, in retrospect, I know that was a mistake. My doctor was flattered that I traveled monthly to Connecticut to see him, but in truth I was terrified of dying from asthma. I firmly believed that I was a severe, steroid-dependent asthmatic who could "check out" at any time. I didn't want to make any treatment changes.

In New York, my asthma didn't get better despite being rabbit-free. Part of the problem was that my lungs were so inflamed after years of abuse that it would take time for them to calm down. My biggest problem, however, was psychological. I accepted my doctor's diagnosis at face value and believed that my life hung by a thread, my only chance for survival being to remain tethered to medication. Adding to my misery was the pressure of pre-medical studies at Columbia and the fact that the steroids were affecting my stomach, keeping me in constant pain. The pain was especially brutal at night, making it difficult to sleep. I even had to visit a gastrointestinal specialist, who placed me on two new medications to protect my stomach from the steroids. I had gained fifty pounds and, by age twenty-seven, was the proud owner of a double chin and a thirty-eight-inch waist.

The real tragedy is that I didn't take steroids because my asthma was severe or because I felt particularly ill. I took steroids because I believed they were keeping me alive. I trusted my doctor when he said I had severe, "difficult to control" asthma and, at the slightest hint of trouble, I should resume steroids to avoid dying. Certain that I constantly teetered on the verge of death, I became emotionally addicted to doctors, medication, and steroids. Yet, as I learned more about asthma, it became increasingly difficult for me to accept my diagnosis. I have always been a "big picture" type of person and, as a doctor, one of the lessons dearest to me is, if you are treating a medical condition that does not respond to standard, high-quality, aggressive therapy, one of two things is probably happening. Either you've misdiagnosed the condition and you're treating the wrong problem, or the condition is worse than you thought.

It troubled me that I was on standard aggressive therapy for years and not getting better. It also bothered me that I never really wheezed or woke up in the middle of the night short of breath, typical complaints for the vast majority of asthmatics. I wheezed when I got sick as a teenager, but beyond that I never had a genuine asthmatic wheeze, even during an "attack." I was also concerned that since I had quit smoking, my asthma didn't flare up when I got a cold. The common cold is notorious for making asthma worse and can often get a previously stable asthmatic into serious trouble. Of equal concern, I knew that nearly every asthmatic feels better on steroids, but that steroids did absolutely nothing for me except make me fat. I had started exercising regularly and couldn't help noticing that my wind was getting better and my peak flow (a measurement used to estimate the severity of asthma) was excellent even during an "attack."

LESSON THREE: ALWAYS GET A SECOND OPINION

One of the problems I have with medicine is the arrogance of some doctors. I hail from New York City, where you tell someone you're a doctor and they shrug their shoulders and say "Yeah, so what?" To me, being a doctor is no big deal. I'm just an average guy who through hard work got himself a good education that led to a decent job. I am no different than other professionals. Unfortunately, there are some physicians who equate being a doctor with being superior. Time for a joke: What is the difference between a doctor and God? God doesn't think he's a doctor. Personally, I would love to be right all the time, but I'm painfully aware that always being right is not part of any doctor's career. Some doctors, however, find it extremely difficult to believe they may be wrong.

I don't know what was going through my doctor's mind, but I do know that, in my practice, when a patient does not respond despite aggressive therapy, I start to wonder whether I'm taking the right approach. I tell the young doctors I train that if they went into medicine expecting everything to be black and white, they're going to be disappointed. More often than doctors care to admit, uncertainty and medicine go hand in hand. Medicine remains a delicate and, at times, a tense balance of science, art, and educated guessing. This is OK. When the patient is getting better and no harm is done, everybody is satisfied. The important lesson I try to convey is, if a patient is not getting better despite appropriate treatment, you will have to reevaluate your diagnosis.

Unfortunately, I suspect my doctor had trouble accepting this basic premise and assumed I had severe asthma. In all fairness to my doctor, after about three years, he did send me for a second opinion to a physician in New York. After the usual history and physical, the New York doctor said, "Well, your doctor is a smart guy, if he says you have asthma, you must have asthma." So, I went back to popping pills and puffing on my inhalers—unbelievable.

Let me share with you the insight I have gained from being both a patient and a physician. Simply stated—there are good doctors and there are bad doctors. I know doctors who I would trust with my life; others I wouldn't let watch my goldfish over the weekend. Nonetheless, the vast majority of doctors are decent, smart people who want to help you get better. I believe it's important to remember that staying healthy requires cooperation between doctor and patient, a partnership that needs the active participation of both parties to achieve a comfortable harmony. In the old days, doctors were only called on when disease had already compromised a person's health. Today, there is an emerging consensus that doctors play only a small role in the healthcare equation and that true health can be found in prevention. An old Chinese proverb says: Superior doctors prevent disease, mediocre doctors treat disease before it is evident, inferior doctors treat full-blown disease.

You need to find a doctor who not only shares this philosophy, but is open to lifestyle modification and so-called alternative or integrative therapy. I say "so-called" because the vitamins, minerals, and herbs that were once considered quackery are increasingly recognized by many medical professionals as possessing healing benefits with scientific validity. You also need to find a doctor you trust and feel comfortable with. A knowledgeable doctor can help you achieve a better understanding of your condition and how it may be influenced by your lifestyle. If, however, you have a physician that does not believe prevention comes before treatment, then perhaps you should consider a new doctor.

While I confess to being a fanatical advocate of prevention and the use of integrative therapies to treat asthma, I do not share the opinion of some alternative healthcare professionals that medication is evil or inherently harmful. Though the goal of this book is to free you of medication, or significantly reduce the amount of medication you use, there will always be some asthmatics who need to be medicated. This is especially true if you have recently been diagnosed with asthma or have poorly controlled asthma. Before you even think about cutting back on your medication, it is vital that you get your asthma under control. Once your asthma is stable, you and your doctor can talk about your medication.

No matter how well or poorly controlled your asthma is right now, you will still benefit tremendously from a careful examinination of your environment and lifestyle in order to make the changes that will ultimately allow you to become medication-free. I want to emphasize that if you've recently been diagnosed with asthma, or your asthma is not stable, then it's important to listen to your physician's advice. The elimination of medication should start when you are stable and feeling your best. Remember, asthma medications help vastly more people than they hurt and only under the most unusual circumstances will these medicines make your asthma worse. If you think your medicine is making your asthma worse and your doctor won't listen, get a second opinion.

Finally, for those asthmatics who land in the emergency room or a hospital bed, this is not the time to experiment or to stop medication. You should have only one mission: to walk out of the hospital alive and well. Once better and stable, I would then question, challenge, and try new strategies.

Back in New York City, I started to wonder if I really had asthma. Sometimes everything comes together at just the right time. As I began to question my diagnosis, two very important things happened in my life. The first occurred early one morning after I stayed up half the night because of stomach pain. I thought to myself, "You're twenty-eight years old, you're overweight, you have stomach pain keeping you up almost every night, you're on numerous medications, one of which is probably doing more harm than good, and you can't leave the house without an inhaler in your pocket. This is no way to live!" I wanted to live, but not like this. I was tired of the fear and pain. When asked if they want to live, most people will nod their heads emphatically and say, "Sure, I want to live." Sounds like an easy question, but it's not. As the decades pass, how willing are you to allow your body to change? How willing are you to give up the activities you enjoyed in your youth? How hard are you willing to work to keep your body fit so you can live a long, healthy life? These are difficult questions and it is not until you see your health being taken away that they hit home.

This is what I mean by "asthma saved my life." I learned at a relatively young age that life is precious and worth living, and that good health cannot be taken for granted. At twenty-eight, I took a good hard look at the way I lived. I saw that the medicines certainly weren't helping and it was time to help myself.

The second important thing that happened was being accepted to medical school, several medical schools actually, and I was torn between New York and Philadelphia. Ultimately, I elected to move to Philadelphia to attend Thomas Jefferson Medical College. This meant that no matter how attached I was to my physician in Connecticut, there was no way I was traveling five hours for a fifteen-minute doctor's appointment.

LESSON FOUR: INSIST ON THE GOLD STANDARD

I shared my doubts about my diagnosis with my new doctor in Philadelphia, who was equally suspicious and ordered a methacholine challenge test. Methacholine is a chemical that causes airway constriction. Everyone reacts to methacholine; asthmatics just have a more intense reaction. The test is considered the gold standard for making a diagnosis of asthma and, in general, the more you react, the more severe your asthma.

My methacholine challenge showed, at worst, mild asthma. Needless to say, I was pleased and not pleased. Not pleased because I wondered why I needed to take so much medicine for six years. I was also concerned about the effect this medication was having on my body, especially my adrenal glands, stomach, and bones. Nor was I terribly happy with the way I looked. The steroids had caused rapid weight gain and stretch marks on several areas of my body—scars that remain with me today.

I was happy because my suspicions were confirmed: my so-called severe asthma was nothing of the sort. I was even happier because all of a sudden that fear of dying a terrible death no longer hung over my head. I was like a man who had just received a death-row pardon. In two months, with the help of my Philadelphia doctor, I was medication-free and slowly losing weight. Most important of all, I felt great!

So, what was going on with my lungs? That's a question that has taken me years to answer. How does someone who allegedly has severe, potentially life-threatening asthma and is steroid-dependent end up diagnosed with only mild asthma and medication-free in two months? I probably had mild asthma since childhood—my asthma was so mild that it only became a problem under the right circumstances, like when I had a cold. This is an extremely important observation. Under the right circumstances, almost anyone can be made to wheeze, and this is especially true of the borderline asthmatic. Also, under the right circumstances, a mild asthmatic can turn into a severe asthmatic.

LESSON FIVE: ASTHMA IS FREQUENTLY AN ENVIRONMENTAL PROBLEM

Many authorities believe that asthma is often an environmental problem. Studies have documented that asthma is relatively rare in non-Western, nonurbanized, sustenance economies. When people move from a society based on a sustenance economy to a more urban area, the incidence of asthma skyrockets. These findings point an accusing finger at environmental insults as a primary factor for much of what we call asthma. I strongly believe that the vast majority of asthmatics can have their asthma "cured," or markedly improved, if they can identify and remove those environmental irritants that are giving them trouble. To this aim, this book is dedicated.

I was (and still am) one of those people with mild asthma who, under the right circumstances, can experience severe disease. Smoking, the common cold, Bumpers the Bunny and his cedar wood chips were all environmental irritants that contributed to kicking my asthma into full gear.

LESSON SIX: RELAX—MAKE ASTHMA THE FIRST STEP TO LASTING HEALTH

Why don't I wheeze? My asthma is an atypical type called "cough variant" asthma, in which instead of wheezing, I cough; this is why I rarely, if ever, wheeze. Why didn't I get better once the rabbit and the smoking were history instead of remaining "sick" for several years? The reason is because I believed I had severe, life-threatening asthma. I was so afraid of dying that I became psychologically addicted to my medications. Every time I felt even a little chest tightness or got a cold, I went right back to the steroids, not wanting to take any chances. Emotionally and physically, I was a prisoner of my disease. I believed my life could be snuffed out at any moment without warning and thought it was better to live in ill health on drugs than be dead.

Moving to Philadelphia was a turning point. Once off the medications, I felt like I had a second chance at life. Having lived under the constant threat of death gave me a new respect for life and living. More important,

I became emotionally free of asthma and this gave me the strength to change my life. I picked up healthy living habits with a vengeance. At forty-two, I'm in the best shape of my life. Nearly every day, I exercise, pushing my lungs and body to their limits. Know what the best part is? My lungs and body respond. Asthma now is no more than an unpleasant footnote to my life, an occasional annoyance. Today, I run, ski, bike, whatever I enjoy doing—and all with impunity. Sure, I occasionally eat ice cream or indulge in a T-bone steak. I'm no culinary monk, but most of the time I treat my body right, and I have remained virtually medication-free for over ten years.

Yet, regardless of how well I feel, I'll always be an asthmatic. But I control my asthma and don't let it control me. In many ways, I am lucky that I was only twenty-three when I learned my diagnosis. I wasn't living healthily and was abusing my body. Having asthma changed me; instead of driving me down, asthma forced me to take control of my life and be responsible for myself. Asthma served as a wake-up call to tell me that my young body was not indestructible, that I was not going to live forever. Asthma made me realize that staying healthy is an active process, one you have to work at every day in a world filled with unhealthy temptations. Asthma is not the first step on a long and bitter road to illness and untimely death—rather, asthma can be the first step to lasting health.

I hope that you're like me and want to live a long and healthy life. Perhaps asthma is a burden to some of you. Perhaps you consider it a slow death sentence. Nothing could be further from the truth. This book will show how asthma can lift you up and give you the meaning, courage, and dedication necessary to live a healthy life.

chapter 1

Relax—You're Not Going to Die of Asthma

MOST PEOPLE WHO SEE A DOCTOR have three basic questions that they rarely, if ever, ask but are always on their minds: "Am I going to die?" "Will I be disabled?" and "How long can I expect to live?" So, let's set the record straight on asthma.

- "Am I going to die?"—No one should die from asthma. The vast majority of asthmatics die at a ripe old age from something else.
- "Will I be disabled?"—Most people with asthma lead normal, physically active lives; at its worst, asthma should only be an occasionally annoying condition.
- "How long can I expect to live?"—Population studies reveal that the overwhelming majority of asthmatics live just as long as anyone else.

ASTHMA CAN BE SCARY

Though reality and statistics are on your side, let's face it, asthma can be scary. Nobody wants to die, especially from an inability to breathe. This lack of breath, this feeling that we can no longer control our body's most basic function, is every asthmatic's nightmare. Without question, asthma is a physical and emotional problem. Walking hand in hand with every medical condition is fear—fear of pain, fear of suffering, fear of death. For most people, this fear is based on half-truths, on misinformation. This is especially true of asthma, where many of us share visions of suffocating through a painful death. But knowledge is power and knowledge about asthma will set you free, allowing you to live the life you deserve.

Let me say this again: There is no reason to die from asthma. As we will see, asthma-related deaths are extraordinarily rare, occurring in less than 1 percent of asthmatics (actually about 0.04 percent). Asthma-related deaths are so rare that they often make sensational newspaper headlines. Let's examine some hard numbers on asthma mortality.

RECENT TRENDS IN ASTHMA

The last twenty-five years have witnessed a staggering increase in the number of people with asthma—we are in the midst of an asthma epidemic. Between 1980 and 1995, the number of new asthma cases in the United States rose over 100 percent for people under eighteen. In 1998, there were approximately 17.3 million asthmatics in the United States (just over 6 percent of the United States population), with an estimated 150 million worldwide. If we look at the number of people who have ever been diagnosed with asthma, the numbers become even more alarming, with 24.7 million people carrying a diagnosis of asthma in 1999. According to the American Lung Association, 10.5 million Americans had an asthma attack or episode in 1999, with 14.6 million Americans experiencing "current asthma" in the year 2000.

No matter how you look at the numbers, it is clear that the number of people with asthma in the United States has risen dramatically in the last quarter of a century. Given this increase in the number of asthmatics, asthma mortality should also rise. Not surprisingly, in 1996 there were 5,667 asthma deaths compared to 2,598 in 1979, a 118 percent increase. The good news is that, thanks to better medications and disease management, this increase in asthma mortality leveled off after 1988 and in 1999 dropped to 4,657 asthma-related deaths (65 percent of which were in women). Another way to look at it: There were on average 1.7 asthma deaths per 100,000 individuals in 1999.

Despite these somewhat reassuring numbers, asthma still exacts a monumental human, social, and economic price. Asthma translates into 10.4 million doctor's office visits, 1.8 million emergency-room visits, and 466,000 hospital admissions. Annually, the economic impact is enormous. Asthma costs in the United States skyrocketed from $6.2 billion in 1990 to $12.7 billion in 2000, with 3 million lost workdays and 10.1 million lost school days.

While asthma is an equal opportunity condition and affects men and women regardless of age or race, some of the greatest increases have, unfortunately, occurred among children. Particularly hard hit are economically disadvantaged children, especially African American children living in poverty. While just over 6 percent of the United States population has asthma, this number increases to over 20 percent in some inner-city schools. A recent study from the Washington University School of Medicine reported that individuals from low socioeconomic areas were 8.4 times more likely to be hospitalized for asthma and 6.4 times more likely to die from asthma. Similar results were found for African Americans in general, who were 5.3 times more likely to be hospitalized for asthma. Equally disturbing, in 1998 asthma prevalence among African American children was 31 percent higher than among Caucasian children. Similar but less dramatic trends were seen in Hispanic children during these same periods.[1]

Authorities blame these numbers on poverty, which acts as a barrier to quality healthcare. Further complicating the plight of the inner city is the lack of air-conditioning, especially during times of high ozone and air pollution levels. Also to blame are high concentrations of cockroaches, which are notorious asthma triggers. Given these considerations, it should come as no surprise that New York City and Chicago are the asthma capitals of America.

WHY THE INCREASE IN ASTHMA?

Even more startling, this asthma epidemic occurred in the shadow of a medical revolution, which gave physicians improved diagnostic and treatment methods. Obviously, this is a cause of concern for physicians, scientists, and public health experts. Many authorities believe that the skyrocketing incidence of asthma can be blamed on oxidant stress. Oxidant stress is a type of daily wear and tear on our cells caused primarily by the environment and the foods we eat. Oxidant stress is blamed for many illnesses, from aging to asthma to heart disease. For asthmatics, one of the most potent sources of oxidant stress is the environment, particularly the air we breathe. Despite tougher emission standards on cars and factories, air pollution remains a major problem for everyone, especially for people who live in cities. Researchers point to increasing levels of ozone, nitrogen dioxide, and sulfur dioxide (gases known to trigger asthma attacks) as the underlying cause of the asthma epidemic.

While outdoor air pollution certainly has had an impact on the asthma epidemic, indoor air pollution is emerging as another major concern. Ever since the energy crisis of the 1970s, new homes are heavily insulated and airtight. Add to this the prevalence of central heating and air-conditioning, combined with synthetic chemical-laden building materials, and it comes as no surprise that indoor levels of air pollution often exceed outdoor levels by several orders of magnitude. While a modest amount of oxidant stress is a normal part of life, there is evidence that our body's defenses are being increasingly overwhelmed by environmental and dietary oxidant stress.

This leads us to the other part of the asthma equation: our diet. Historically, our chief defense against oxidant stress has been natural dietary antioxidants. Unfortunately, we are eating fewer antioxidant-rich foods like fresh fruits and vegetables and consuming more oxidant-heavy foods like animal fat and junk food. In fact, studies have shown that many asthmatics are deficient in several vital antioxidant vitamins and minerals. It is this decreased dietary antioxidant intake coupled with increased environmental oxidant stress that many believe is responsible for the asthma epidemic.

WHO DIES FROM ASTHMA?

Traditionally, the asthmatic at greatest risk of dying is the "brittle asthmatic," who has repeated life-threatening asthma attacks despite aggressive medical treatment. Over the past twenty-five years, we have seen a jump in deaths among non-brittle asthmatics. These deaths are largely confined to females over the age of sixty-five. Because they make up such a large proportion of the American population, white female asthmatics, age sixty-five and over, accounted for most of the increase in the rate of asthma-related deaths. African American female asthmatics over the age of sixty-five, however, had the most rapid increase in overall rate of asthma-related deaths between 1979 and 1996.

When adjusted for age, the greatest increase in asthma-related deaths occurred in black females age sixty-five and older, followed by black males over sixty-five, then white females in the same age group, and finally black females thirty-four to sixty-four years old.[2] In a study on near-fatal asthma attacks in Washington, DC, researchers at George Washington University Medical Center found that 84 percent of the subjects were African Americans. Equally disturbing was the author's conclusion that "up to one third of the events may have been preventable."[3] Viewed another way, the death rate among African Americans was three times higher than among Caucasians, with 3.9 asthma deaths per 100,000 African Americans (4.2 deaths per 100,000 African American women). It has been a very tough twenty-five years for asthmatics in the African American community.

An alarming finding from these studies is how illegal drugs and alcohol contribute to asthma mortality. Researchers at Northwestern University Medical School, in Chicago, Illinois, examined forty-two cases of asthma-related deaths and found that 38 percent of these individuals tested positive for illegal drugs.[4] Other studies report that up to 60 percent of asthma-related deaths can be traced back to alcohol or illegal drugs like cocaine, PCP (phencyclidine or angel dust), and morphine. I am continually amazed that asthmatics would risk their health, even their lives, in such a way. Clearly, alcohol and drug addiction is a serious problem for anyone, but it can be fatal to an asthmatic. Avoiding serious asthma trouble is simple: Don't smoke, don't use illegal drugs or abuse alcohol, eat a healthy diet, exercise, and develop a good relationship with your doctor. That's all you have to do!

Finally, advanced age appears to be another risk factor for asthma-related death. According to the American Lung Association, asthma deaths increase with age, with the highest death rate found in individuals eighty-five years and older. In 1999, there were 17.2 asthma-related deaths per 100,000 individuals in this age group.

The encouraging news is that deaths from asthma have leveled off since 1988 and even declined, thanks in large part to improved disease management. Statistics from the American Lung Association indicate that asthma-related deaths declined 3 percent in 1999 with a 7.4 percent decrease in the asthma attack rate between 1997 and 1999.

To sum up, what are some of the risk factors for asthma-related death?

- Female age sixty-five and over
- African American
- Low income
- Low education
- Drug or alcohol abuse
- Advanced age

There is one thing I want to make perfectly clear: No one should die from asthma. Even if you're reading this list and shaking your head because you have one or more risk factors, by gathering information about your condition, you may have just saved your life. Arming yourself with knowledge will enable you to control your asthma no matter how much money you make or how much education you have. The information in this book is for everyone—black, white, male, female, young, old, rich, poor, and everyone in between. The lessons learned in this book will not only help you beat asthma but will help you in all areas of your life, empowering you to take control of your health.

Clear-cut lists are convenient, but asthma mortality is more complicated. The reality is that life-saving health information and quality healthcare rarely find their way to the inner city. While low education may often translate into low income, the real problem is when people are woefully misinformed about health and are placed in double jeopardy because they cannot afford professional advice.

Picking up a book on asthma, and showing concern about your health, in and of itself dramatically reduces your risk for having a serious asthma problem. Clearly, reaching less fortunate populations is a major challenge for public health experts. The real reason people die from asthma is because they don't understand the condition and lack access to healthcare providers who can offer them knowledge and quality care.

BEYOND THE STATISTICS: ATTITUDE AND OTHER FACTORS

I hope you feel better about your risk of dying from asthma. The truth is, if you treat your body with respect, your asthma should be no more than a minor footnote to an otherwise healthy and active life. Understanding why people die from asthma can calm your fears and help you avoid the mistakes that cause asthmatics trouble. We have already learned that, statistically speaking, the people most likely to die from asthma are women age sixty-five and over. Many of you are probably saying, "I'm not a woman nor am I over sixty-five, so what's my risk?"

Perhaps the most important risk factor for asthma trouble is attitude. The vast majority of people I've seen die from asthma really died from self-neglect. Sure, it was their lungs that ultimately did them in, but most of these people were abusing their lungs. For instance, many people with asthma smoke. There is no question that smoking makes your asthma dramatically worse and nearly impossible to control. Asthmatics who smoke are the ones I see every week in the emergency room for their "severe asthma," which, if they behaved rationally (that is, didn't smoke), would probably only be mild or moderate asthma. These same asthmatics may one day end up in the intensive care unit, or dead.

Equally troubling are the asthmatics who would rather be sick than give up their pet. If an asthmatic is allergic to cats but insists on keeping Fi Fi, it's easy to figure out why they're in the emergency room every week. While asthmatics are no doubt emotionally attached to their pets just like other pet owners, they need to be aware of the detrimental health consequences in keeping a pet. Moral of the story: Don't smoke, and think critically about keeping your pets.

Another group I commonly see getting into trouble are the people who deny they have asthma or do not take their asthma seriously. These are often the same people who refuse to exercise, skip doctor appointments, and live on fatty and fast foods. There are also asthmatics who place too much trust in their doctors, expecting that taking a pill or inhaling some medicine will make their asthma disappear. As we will learn, this attitude can be just as dangerous as ignoring asthma. One theme I will stress repeatedly in this book is that healthcare is a two-way street and that medicine should play only a small role for the vast majority of asthmatics. The key to beating asthma is preventing your lungs from acting up in the first place.

Also increasing your risk for asthma trouble is the number of times you've been in the emergency room (ER) for asthma. The average number of emergency-room visits for asthma is 1.8 million annually. If you have never been in an ER for your asthma, this means your condition is probably mild to moderate, relatively well controlled, and your chances of having a serious problem are very slim. In other words, your asthma may annoy you, but you'll probably never die from it.

A history of multiple ER trips for asthma, however, indicates that a person has severe asthma that is difficult to control, or has poorly controlled mild to moderate asthma. The same can be said for multiple hospital admissions. A history of intubation—meaning that a person's asthma was so severe that they needed to be placed on a ventilator so they could breathe—is another major risk factor. Being intubated translates into severe or poorly controlled asthma; one study found that people who had a history of mechanical ventilation were twenty-seven times more likely to experience near-fatal asthma. Likewise, having been admitted to the intensive care unit (ICU) is a potent risk factor; the study on intubation also found that a history of ICU admission increased near-fatal asthma risk by ten times.[5]

THE REASONS WHY YOU ARE NOT GOING TO DIE FROM ASTHMA

People with asthma really die from denial and neglect—their lungs are just innocent bystanders. By reading this book, you are taking important steps that may save your life. You have decided that it is time to learn more about your asthma and you now realize that asthma is a problem that must be addressed. The simple truth is that the more you know about your condition, the more control you have over it. This is true if you have asthma, diabetes, heart disease, or any other medical problem. The vast majority of asthma trouble is seen in people who deny they have a problem or lack the knowledge to take care of their asthma.

If you live your life right, exercise, eat a healthy diet, establish a trusting relationship with a good doctor, you're not going to die from asthma. After studying why people die from asthma, three fundamental truths emerge:

1. The vast majority of asthma deaths are preventable.
2. People don't die from asthma, they die from denial and ignorance.
3. You really have to work hard to die from asthma. Remember, less than 1 percent of asthmatics die because of it.

ASTHMA AND DISABILITY

Regarding the second question—"Will I be disabled?"—much of this book answers the question by showing you how to stay physically and mentally fit so you can control your life. In fact, the real question for asthmatics concerns not disability but ability: What do you want to *do?* The answer will vary from person to person and this book will help you arrive at a conclusion that suits you best. We'll talk more about asthma and athletic excellence in Chapter 5, but there are no limits when it comes to ability and the asthmatic. Some of you may be surprised to learn that approximately 15 percent of the 1996 Summer Olympics athletes in Atlanta had asthma. Almost 50 percent of the cycling and mountain-biking Olympic team members reported a history of asthma.[6]

ASTHMA AND LIFE EXPECTANCY

Unlike people with heart disease, diabetes, or cancer, asthma has no impact on life expectancy for the overwhelming majority of people. Also, unlike other diseases that can result in permanent and, at times, lethal organ damage, asthma leaves the lungs relatively intact. You may have heard that asthma causes irreversible lung damage. While this is true for a minority of asthmatics, these people usually have a lung condition like emphysema that is responsible for the damage; there is no evidence that asthma by itself causes lung damage. As long as you avoid other risk factors such as smoking or alcohol/drug abuse, your lungs can remain relatively healthy with asthma.

According to *Harrison's Principles of Internal Medicine,* the "bible" of internal medicine for most physicians, the typical lifetime course of asthma is as follows: Even when untreated, individuals with asthma do not continuously move from mild to severe disease with time. Rather, their clinical course is characterized by exacerbations and remissions. Some studies suggest that spontaneous remissions occur in approximately 20 percent of those who develop the disease as adults and that 40 percent or so can be expected to experience improvement, with less frequent and severe attacks, as they grow older.[7]

The news is even better for children with asthma. According to *Harrison's,* the number of children who still have asthma seven to ten years after the initial diagnosis varies from 26 percent to 78 percent, averaging 46 percent; however, the percentage of children who continue to have severe disease is relatively low, 6 to 19 percent.[8]

Several major studies have specifically examined the impact asthma has on life expectancy. One recent study from the Mayo Clinic, published in *The New England Journal of Medicine,* examined the life expectancy of 2,499 asthmatics. The study followed these asthmatics for fourteen to twenty-nine years, and the authors concluded that survival among patients with asthma but no other lung disease was not significantly different from expected survival. The study did find that asthmatics with another medical condition, like emphysema, "have worse than expected survival."[9] This is not surprising, since smoking is the leading cause of emphysema and it's no secret that smoking and longevity don't mix.

I hope this chapter has made it clear that you're not going to die from asthma and that asthma will not affect how long you do the cha-cha, participate in athletic activities, or do anything else! Not only can you lead a normal and physically demanding life, but you can actually win the war against asthma. To beat asthma, it helps to first understand exactly what asthma is. So, let's take a crash course on the physiology of asthma.

chapter 2

Asthma Basics

"WHAT IS ASTHMA?" If you can answer this question to everyone's satisfaction, you just may get a Nobel Prize. The most common definition considers asthma a chronic inflammatory disorder characterized by episodes of reversible bronchospasm, commonly known as an asthma attack. If you pick up a standard medical dictionary and look up the word "asthma," you'll probably read something like this: "Asthma is a chronic inflammatory disease of the airways that is characterized by increased responsiveness of the tracheobronchial tree to a multiplicity of stimuli."[1]

In less technical jargon, asthma is a medical condition that affects the lung's airways, causing them to become smaller and thereby blocking airflow. This airway obstruction is reversible, meaning the blockage eventually goes away, either by itself or through the use of medication. Doctors call this airway constriction "bronchospasm" or "bronchoconstriction." What causes this reversible bronchoconstriction varies from person to person and can range from allergies to exercise to emotions. Central to bronchospasm is a chronic inflammation of the airways that makes them more sensitive and more likely to constrict under the right circumstances. Why asthmatics have this chronic inflammation and why asthma varies from person to person are questions subject to intense controversy. Still confused? So are a lot of scientists and physicians. Perhaps the best way to view asthma is to consider it as several different problems rolled into one, with environmental, allergic, genetic, emotional, infectious, and nutritional factors, along with immune dysfunction, each playing a role.

WHY DO PEOPLE GET ASTHMA?

"Why do I have asthma?" The answer to this question varies from person to person. We do know that virtually every asthmatic has hyperreactive airways, but the real question is "Why?" There is an emerging consensus that asthma results from a complex interplay between genes and environment, that people who have inherited particular genes will develop asthma if exposed to the proper environment. Genetic analysis has made it increasingly clear that many genes are responsible for asthma. We presently can't control our genetic heritage, but as gene therapy matures we may one day be able to genetically treat asthma along with many other medical disorders, from diabetes to cancer.

Though we can't control our genes, we can control our environment. Environment has become increasingly recognized as a major contributor to asthma. Many people can have their asthma "cured" if they can identify and remove the appropriate environmental triggers. This is supported by numerous studies that place responsibility for the current asthma epidemic on our urbanized, Western culture. Population studies have found that asthma is primarily a problem of affluent, industrialized societies. In fact, asthma is rare in many of the world's poorest countries. One study, published in *The Lancet,* examined the incidence of asthma in Ethiopia and found that urban children were three times more likely to have asthma than rural children, an effect the authors attributed to "general changes in the domestic environment."[2] Another study found that the incidence of asthma in urban South Africa was 3.17 percent compared to only 0.14 percent in a rural area.[3]

What is responsible for this geographic variation is the million-dollar question. As you can imagine, when you get a group of physicians and scientists in the same room to discuss the causes of asthma, you get some lively controversy. The general consensus is that the asthma epidemic results from a combination of dietary and environmental factors, most notably oxidant stress. Throughout this book we will carefully examine these dietary and environmental factors, offering advice on how you can avoid these asthma triggers.

ANATOMY OF THE LUNG 101

Before we continue talking about asthma, it may help if we understand a little more about what a lung is and what it does. The body's cells need oxygen to survive; once the cells use the oxygen, they make carbon dioxide, a cellular waste product. The lung's primary job is to bring oxygen into the body, where it is absorbed by the blood. The blood carries the oxygen to the cells and takes away the carbon dioxide, which is brought to the lungs where it is exhaled. To exchange gases efficiently with the bloodstream requires a large surface area—the lungs are perfectly suited for this job, having a surface area roughly the size of a football field.

The air people breathe through the nose or mouth travels through the trachea, the main airway that feeds the lungs. The trachea divides into two main stem bronchi, one for each lung, which in turn subdivide into smaller and smaller intrapulmonary bronchi that deliver air to different parts of the lungs. These bronchi ultimately subdivide into even smaller bronchioles, which are divided into "terminal" and "respiratory" bronchioles. The respiratory bronchioles lead to alveolar ducts that become the alveoli. It is primarily at the level of the alveoli that oxygen enters the blood and carbon dioxide leaves the blood.

BRONCHOCONSTRICTION AND INCREASED AIRWAY RESPONSIVENESS

Asthmatic bronchoconstriction is usually constriction of the medium- to small-sized airways. This constriction occurs in part because the muscle that surrounds a lung's airways contracts during an asthma attack, thereby obstructing airflow and increasing the work of breathing. This increased effort is perceived by an asthmatic as an uncomfortable "chest tightness" or "air hunger." Adding to the airflow obstruction is the fact that the asthmatic's airways are normally filled with mucus that is thicker and more abundant than normal.

Increased airway responsiveness is perhaps the most important feature of asthma. To understand exactly what increased airway "responsiveness" means, we have to understand that the airways of all people, both those with and without asthma, can constrict if exposed to certain stimuli. For instance, most people will have mild airway narrowing after exposure to agents known to cause bronchoconstriction, like methacholine, ozone, or histamine. Asthmatics, however, after exposure to any of these agents, tend to experience more pronounced airway narrowing when compared to non-asthmatics. Not only are asthmatics more responsive to agents known to cause bronchoconstriction, but the airways of an asthmatic often constrict after exposure to agents that normal airways would not react to at all.

For instance, asthmatics can have an attack after being exposed to certain smells, wood dust, allergens, and so on—the list is nearly endless.

CHRONIC INFLAMMATION AND FREE RADICALS

In addition to increased airway reactivity, the lungs of an asthmatic are usually chronically inflamed. Even when we microscopically examine an asthmatic's lungs between attacks, we find inflammatory cells surrounding the airways. An inflammatory cell works with the immune system to fight infection and tissue injury. There are various types of inflammatory cells, including eosinophils, lymphocytes, mast cells, macrophages, and neutrophils. They release chemicals such as histamine, prostaglandins, bradykinin, interferon, and endothelin-1 that work together to kill fungi, bacteria, and viruses. Perhaps the most important cells in asthma are the T cells (T lymphocytes), especially the CD4+ Th2 subset, which researchers say plays a pivotal role in the immune system abnormalities seen in asthma. Researchers believe that a shift in the balance from Th1 to Th2 is a leading cellular mechanism in asthma, because increased Th2 levels result in elevated levels of leukotrienes, prostaglandin E_2, and certain interleukins—chemical mediators known to initiate and perpetuate inflammation and asthma.

Most of these chemicals, besides killing germs, are known to be potent instigators of bronchoconstriction. For reasons that remain poorly understood, asthmatic lungs are chronically on the defensive, always ready to fight and release these inflammatory mediators at the slightest provocation. Ironically, the same cells that are intended to protect us can actually cause harm in the asthmatic.

This is how the immune response works: A bacterium enters the lungs and is recognized by the immune system. The immune system sounds the alarm for the inflammatory cells to come rushing in to release chemicals and free radicals that kill the invading bacteria. Free radicals are highly reactive oxygen molecules that cause such profound damage to the germ that it dies. Free radicals are used by our immune system to kill invading organisms.

The only problem is that when these free radicals are released, they kill not only the invading organism but also some surrounding normal tissue, a kind of shotgun approach to healing. Usually, this is not a problem since only a tiny amount of healthy tissue is damaged and the body can repair itself. Then, after the bug is killed, the inflammatory cells calm down and the immune system returns to normal. Sure, a few inflammatory cells will remain to watch the fort, but after the battle is over most of the cells depart.

In asthmatics, these inflammatory cells never calm down and stay in the lung. Even worse, they continue as if the fight isn't over, spewing out toxic chemicals and free radicals that damage the lungs. Like toxic chemicals, free radicals are potent bronchoconstrictors and there is evidence that the free radicals produced by asthmatics are more reactive than normal. One French study concluded, "there was a significant correlation between the overall severity of asthma and the amount of reactive species of oxygen generated."[4] So what you have in the asthmatic is a state of chronic inflammation that promotes bronchoconstriction.

Chronic inflammation and tissue damage makes water enter the lungs. This is called pulmonary edema. The more water in the lungs, the more narrow the airways become and the greater the airway obstruction. Add to this the fact that inflammatory cells tend to recruit more inflammatory cells and you have a self-perpetuating cycle of airway inflammation, tissue damage, and edema. Making matters worse, these chemicals cause the lungs to make more mucus that, in turn, further obstructs the airway.

These chemicals and free radicals also gang up on the cells that line the airways, the epithelial cells. The epithelium is designed to protect the lungs; however, in asthma, the epithelium gets tricked by the inflammatory cells into thinking the lung is under attack and releases its own chemicals that help perpetuate this vicious cycle. This further damages the airway epithelium, which ultimately falls off, leaving behind raw lung tissue that can no longer defend itself. Doctors suspect that once this protective epithelium is removed, nerve endings are exposed causing the nerves to send panic signals to the rest of the lung, resulting in widespread bronchoconstriction, inflammation, and edema—otherwise known as an asthmatic attack.

So, in asthma, there are too many inflammatory cells that, instead of protecting the lungs, actually harm them by constantly generating toxic chemicals and free radicals. These chemicals and free radicals injure the lung's epithelial lining, resulting in both increased airway reactivity and bronchospasm.

While all this sounds pretty grim, the good news is that many natural therapies are designed to reduce the state of chronic inflammation. What this means for you is better control of your symptoms. And there's more good news. Free radicals cause lung damage by a mechanism called "oxidative stress." Under normal circumstances, our bodies are able to neutralize this oxidative stress with natural antioxidants like vitamins C and E. In asthma, our natural antioxidant defenses become overwhelmed, ultimately resulting in bronchoconstriction. However, we can boost our antioxidant defenses naturally through diet and supplements, breaking this cycle.

ASTHMA SYMPTOMS

The unhappy marriage between increased airway responsiveness and chronic inflammation causes periodic narrowing of the airways that we call an asthma attack. In general, the more the airways narrow, the worse the attack. Most people describe an asthma attack as a sensation of "air hunger" or "chest tightness," as if they can't get enough air into their lungs. However, the converse is actually true; people with asthma cannot get enough air out of their lungs. This is because airway narrowing obstructs airflow and prevents air from leaving the lungs, a process called "air trapping." People with asthma feel like they can't get enough air because the trapped old air is filling up the lung and not leaving enough room for the fresh air to get in.

One of the hallmarks of asthma is that between attacks, the vast majority of asthmatics feel fine. Asthma is an episodic condition characterized by occasional attacks interspersed by symptom-free periods that can range from hours or days to months or years. The fact that asthma comes and goes often presents a challenge to physicians, since it is difficult to establish a diagnosis of asthma unless the person is having symptoms. This is why some asthmatics wait months or years before a physician will commit to a diagnosis of asthma.

Attacks are usually accompanied by variable amounts of wheezing that can range from so fine that it can only be heard through a stethoscope to wheezing that can be heard across the room. Coughing is another symptom commonly reported by asthmatics. In fact, some asthmatics never wheeze and instead, their chief complaint is a chronic, nonproductive (dry) cough. This type of asthma is called "cough-variant asthma" (the type of asthma I have). Some people only have asthma symptoms following exercise, which is known as "exercise-induced asthma." Many asthmatics will also tell you that their symptoms are worse at night. It is not uncommon to find an asthmatic who awakens short of breath in the middle of the night or early in the morning.

Asthma attacks usually evolve gradually over a period of minutes, and the classic allergic asthma attack can be divided into an early and late phase. The early phase is characterized by bronchoconstriction and produces the symptoms traditionally associated with asthma. This phase usually lasts for thirty to sixty minutes and is often described as "chest tightness" that is frequently accompanied by a dry cough. Wheezing, if present, may be initially heard only during expiration, but if the constriction becomes moderate to severe, wheezing may be audible during expiration and inspiration. Heart and respiratory rates often increase as breathing becomes more difficult; some asthmatics sweat or experience anxiety during an attack. Most asthmatics know when an attack is over and feel fine almost immediately afterwards. For many asthmatics, the end of an attack is often heralded by a dry cough that turns into a productive cough generating thick, stringy mucus. Surprisingly, however, though an asthmatic may tell you that an attack is over, studies have shown that impaired lung function can persist for hours or days after an attack.

The second phase of an allergic asthma attack occurs approximately three to eight hours after the first phase and is also characterized by airway obstruction. Unlike the first phase, airway obstruction in the second phase is caused by inflammation and edema. These two phases of the allergic asthmatic response have implications for the conventional medical management of asthma. This is in part why standard medical therapy includes albuterol and inhaled steroids. Bronchodilators like albuterol are often used to treat the initial bronchoconstriction, whereas anti-inflammatory steroids are used to treat the inflammatory phase. These phases also have profound implications for natural asthma remedies, a subject covered in Chapters 7 and 8. As you will learn, not only do many natural remedies have bronchodilatory and anti-inflammatory effects, but many are also directed toward prevention and boosting the body's natural antioxidant defenses.

One of the best lessons you can learn is that most doctors would be hard-pressed to find two asthmatics whose symptoms and triggers are exactly alike. Asthma symptoms and severity vary markedly from person to person, and the list of potential asthma triggers is virtually endless. A "typical" asthma attack can last from minutes to hours to days. Some people have multiple daily attacks, whereas others have symptoms only once or twice a month. Some people have symptoms year-round, while others have allergy-related asthma that only acts up during the spring or fall.

Some asthmatics have very mild asthma, while others have unpredictable and unusually severe attacks. The majority of asthmatics fall somewhere in between these two extremes, with most asthma attacks ranging from mild to moderate.

HOW DO YOU KNOW IF YOU'RE HAVING A SEVERE ASTHMA ATTACK?

Despite the almost endless variation among asthmatics, the overwhelming majority of people with asthma have mild to moderate asthma that is predictable. While it is also true that, under the right circumstances, even a person with mild asthma can have a severe attack, most asthmatics will never experience such an attack. Equally assuring, the typical asthmatic can look forward to their symptoms becoming less severe over time. This is especially true for those individuals who learn about and take care of their asthma.

Still, everyone should know the warning signs of a severe or a potentially severe asthma attack. One of the first and strongest warning signs is how the asthmatic feels. For most asthmatics, their symptoms are often predictable and one attack doesn't vary much from the last. Most asthmatics can tell if they're getting better or getting worse. So, the first sign that trouble may be on the horizon is that your symptoms are getting worse. Another warning sign is when your symptoms don't respond to the usual treatment that, in the past, tended to put an end to an attack.

Another danger signal is nasal flaring, meaning that the soft bottom sides of your nose move out away from the midline as you breathe. Nasal flaring is usually only seen during a moderate to severe attack and indicates increased trouble breathing. Asthmatics with a severe (potentially life-threatening) attack may have difficulty speaking in full sentences and may only be able to say two or three words at a time. More severe attacks are characterized by an inability to speak with or without accessory muscle use. The accessory muscles, like the neck or chest muscles, help people breathe during a severe attack. You can tell someone is using accessory muscles if they shrug their shoulders as they breathe or if their breathing appears labored.

During a life-threatening attack, the wheezing may become high-pitched or even disappear. An asthmatic who stops wheezing while still short of breath is an asthmatic in serious trouble. Wheezing is caused by bronchoconstriction that partially obstructs, but does not completely prevent, airflow. When an asthmatic stops wheezing, it means one of two things: the asthma attack is over, or the person has stopped moving air through his or her lungs.

Life-threatening attacks can also cause cyanosis, or turning blue. Cyanosis is an ominous sign and means there is a profound lack of oxygen in the blood, a condition known as hypoxia. Hypoxia is extremely dangerous because the less oxygen the blood has, the less it can deliver to vital organs like the brain and heart. Stated bluntly, hypoxia is what kills asthmatics.

Fortunately, such severe attacks are extremely rare. However, if you or a loved one is having an attack and appears drowsy, is gasping for air, starts to turn blue, or stops wheezing without feeling better, do not hesitate to call 911—this is a medical emergency.

If you find yourself in the emergency room for an asthma attack, I strongly recommend taking full advantage of modern medicine. You may not be happy receiving steroids and other drugs, but if your symptoms are so severe that you land in the hospital, your first priority should be getting better and leaving the hospital alive. Once stable, you can learn from what happened and make sure it doesn't happen again.

PHYSIOLOGICAL RISK FACTORS FOR ASTHMA

The risk factors for asthma remain poorly understood, but it appears that asthma results from a combination of genetic and environmental factors. The strongest risk factor for asthma is atopy, an exaggerated response to the environment. In other words, the lungs of asthmatics tend to respond more intensely to stimuli like cat dander or wood dust. Atopy frequently runs in families, and people with asthma often have allergies or family members with asthma and/or allergies. The allergic reactions found in people with atopy can range from seasonal hay fever to eczema to asthma. People with atopy also have increased blood levels of immunoglobulin E (IgE), the chief mediator of allergic and asthmatic reactions. In fact, IgE plays such a critical role in asthma that, in general, the higher the IgE level, the more severe the asthma.

Without question, asthma runs in families; however, there are many asthmatics who do not have a family history of allergies or asthma. The claim that asthma most likely results from a combination of genetic and environmental factors means that some people are genetically more prone to develop asthma and will display symptoms if exposed to the proper environment. It appears that several genetic abnormalities are involved in asthma, which may, in part, explain the extreme variability among asthmatics.

Another major risk factor for asthma is exposure to tobacco smoke, especially as a child. Numerous studies have documented that children raised in the homes of smokers have a significantly increased risk of lung problems, especially asthma. Living near freeways or in large cities may also increase asthma risk, as several studies have shown a link between air pollution and the risk of lung disease.

Some researchers suspect that being first-born increases risk, whereas coming from a large family may actually decrease risk. Why this is true remains a mystery and is the subject of intense research. It is also suspected that certain respiratory tract infections in childhood can increase the risk of developing asthma later in life. Finally, emotions and asthma often go hand in hand. One study, which followed 5,231 adults for thirteen years, found that anxiety and depression increased the risk of developing asthma dramatically.[5]

It is important to divide risk factors into those we can and those we cannot control. While many risk factors are beyond our control, whether or not you smoke and what you eat can be controlled. As you will read later in this book, what we eat does have a profound impact on our health. And in Chapter 7, multiple nutrient deficiencies are identified as asthma risk factors.

TYPES OF ASTHMA

It is convenient to divide asthma into several subtypes. These subtypes may be somewhat artificial, since most asthmatics share several features of each subtype, but these distinctions help to better understand and treat asthma. Asthma is generally divided into "idiosyncratic" and "stimuli evoked."

"Idiosyncratic" means we don't know what caused the attack. True idiosyncratic asthma is rare, so what this name usually implies is that we haven't discovered what provoked the attack. "Stimuli evoked" means that the asthma attack was caused by exposure to a particular stimulus. The substances that can cause an attack are almost endless, ranging from pollen to cold air. It is convenient to divide stimuli-evoked asthma into different categories: allergic, infectious, emotional, drug- or food-related, environmental, occupational or work-related, exercise-induced, and gastroesophageal reflux-associated asthma. Further complicating matters is that there is a significant degree of overlap between the two primary categories of asthma, with some people one day clearly having stimuli-evoked asthma and on another day experiencing an attack for no apparent reason.

Idiosyncratic Asthma

For some asthmatics, we cannot readily determine what's triggering their asthma, despite extensive testing. These asthmatics are called "idiopathic" or "idiosyncratic." True idiopathic asthma is becoming a rarity as we learn more and more about asthma. For most idiopathic asthmatics, time, coupled with some detective work, will ultimately reveal what triggers their attacks.

Conventional and Integrative Approach—Extensive testing, asthma diary review, and complete evaluation of home and work environments is needed to identify offending agents. The conventional approach uses medications like albuterol and inhaled steroids to manage symptoms. As you will learn in later chapters, the integrative approach employs a variety of natural remedies and non-pharmacological treatments to reduce bronchoconstriction and inflammation.

Allergic Asthma

In allergic asthma an allergen, such as dust, pollen, or cat dander, is triggering the attack. It is estimated that 50 to 80 percent of asthmatics have an allergic component to their asthma. What triggers the attack varies from person to person and can change over time; however, most of these allergens are airborne. Inhaled allergens are potent triggers in susceptible individuals and can produce an immediate asthmatic response that may be followed by several weeks of increased airway reactivity. Many people who develop asthma from airborne allergens at first require large amounts of allergen to provoke a reaction. Over time, as the person becomes sensitized, smaller and smaller amounts of the offending allergen are needed to trigger a response.

Many people with allergic asthma only have symptoms during a particular time of the year, such as the spring when pollen counts are high. In fact, when there are high pollen counts, hospitals frequently record elevated numbers of asthma-related emergency-room visits and deaths. Other people can exhibit allergic asthma year-round if they happen to be allergic to stimuli like animals, feathers, or dust mites.

Most people with allergic asthma have an almost immediate reaction to the offending allergen, called the "acute response." Approximately 30 to 50 percent of acute responders will experience a "late response" six to ten hours later. Some people never experience the acute response and only develop the late response to a particular allergen. As with most asthma triggers, the best way to treat allergic asthma is to avoid the allergen. We'll talk more about allergen-trigger avoidance in Chapter 6.

Conventional Approach—I recommend allergy testing for every asthmatic. While no test is perfect, allergy testing can alert you to potential allergens. Tests can range from the simple "scratch-and-prick" to intradermal injections to more elaborate allergy testing. Talk to your doctor about which testing method is best for you. If you can't avoid an allergen, like pollen, there are many excellent, non-sedating antihistamines available (ask your doctor).

Integrative Approach—Once again, formal allergy testing is indicated. Knowing your enemy will help you avoid it. Many natural remedies for allergy sufferers are available and range from vitamin C to the herb *ma huang*. For an extensive discussion on integrative medicine and allergies, see Chapters 7 and 8 or the *User's Guide to Natural Allergy Relief* (Basic Health Publications, 2003).

Infectious Asthma

If anything gets an asthmatic in trouble, it's a viral infection. In fact, viral infections are perhaps the most common triggers of an asthma exacerbation and some asthmatics only have symptoms during and after a cold. This is why I constantly harp on getting enough sleep, exercise, and eating a healthy diet. Not so you look good naked, which isn't a bad thing, but so your immune system stays strong to fight viral infections. Parainfluenza and respiratory syncytial viruses cause the most trouble for children, whereas influenza and rhinovirus are the usual suspects in adults. Rhinovirus is the bug often responsible for the common cold. Viral infections cause damage by increasing airway inflammation and sensitivity, which in turn can worsen asthmatic symptoms for weeks to months.

Conventional Approach—Good old-fashioned prevention and healthy living is the best remedy. Treatment relies primarily on relief of symptoms, with acetaminophen for fever and pain coupled with liberal bed rest and fluids.

Integrative Approach—As in Western methods, prevention is the key. One to two grams of vitamin C daily may help you avoid the common cold.

Emotional Asthma

While allergies and infections have traditionally shared the blame for the vast majority of asthma attacks, emotions have increasingly been recognized as playing a major role. Attitudes and emotions can cut both ways, making or breaking your asthma. It's good news for asthma control if you have a positive attitude, bad news if you have a negative attitude. It is estimated that half of all asthmatics have an emotional component to their condition. Some individuals can make their symptoms better or worse just by thinking about them. There are even a few asthmatics who can consciously modify their airway response to inhaled stimuli.

I know from personal experience that the more I worry about my asthma, the worse it tends to become. I also know that I can have an asthma attack just from thinking or reading about asthma. When I was asked to write this book, I was a "closet" asthmatic. Despite a rocky beginning in my twenties, by the age of forty I rarely had an attack and was essentially medication-free. Writing this book once again forced me to come face-to-face with my asthma, and for two months I had some trouble; I even had to use a short course of inhaled steroids. Other asthmatics can be enslaved by a vicious cycle of fear and anxiety. In fact, there is increasing evidence that emotions figure prominently in the potentially lethal asthma subtype known as brittle asthma. For better or worse, in many ways we are what we think. To learn more about asthma and emotions, see Chapter 9.

Conventional Approach—I recommend avoiding antianxiety and antidepressant medications unless all other less invasive approaches have failed. While these medications certainly play a vital and appropriate role in the lives of many people, they are treatments of last resort.

Integrative Approach—This can range from yoga to biofeedback to psychotherapy. Whatever eases your anxiety and, most important, works. To learn more about this therapy, read Chapter 9.

Drug- and Food-Related Asthma

Almost any drug can cause an asthma attack in a susceptible individual; however, the most common offenders are aspirin and beta-blockers. Beta-blockers are medications commonly used for glaucoma, high blood pressure, and heart problems. They are given to asthmatics only under the most unusual of circumstances. Aspirin is a notorious and potentially dangerous asthma trigger, especially in individuals with nasal polyps. Other common medicines that can cause trouble for asthmatics are nonsteroidal, anti-inflammatory drugs (NSAIDs), such as ibuprofen. Included in this group are over-the-counter agents like Advil, Aleve, Motrin, and naproxen. It is believed that NSAIDs exacerbate asthma by blocking cyclooxygenase, leading to increased leukotriene production.

Drug allergies are especially dangerous for the asthmatic since medications are taken internally where they can have a maximal effect, in rare instances causing death. This does not mean that asthmatics can't take these medications. Only about 10 percent of asthmatics are allergic to aspirin; I have personally used aspirin and NSAIDs for years without trouble. Acetaminophen (Tylenol) usually does not cause problems for asthmatics. Most of you probably know by now what medicines and foods you can eat and those you cannot. If you've been taking ibuprofen without any problems for the last twenty years, now is not the time to stop. If, however, you have never taken aspirin, now is not the time to start. If in doubt, check with your doctor to see if the medicine you are taking (or about to take) is safe.

Food allergies can be caused by the food itself or by something artificial in the food, like a food coloring or preservative. Food colorings are used virtually everywhere, so it's important to read food and drug labels to see if food coloring is present. Sulfiting agents, another common allergy trigger, are used as preservatives in medicines and food. Common sulfiting agents include potassium bisulfite, potassium metabisulfite, sodium bisulfite, sodium sulfite, and sulfur dioxide. Sulfites can hide anywhere, from the salad bar to your favorite wine, and are even present in some asthma medications, like intravenous steroids and inhaled agents. This, in part, explains why you hear about the rare asthmatic who gets worse with treatment. If you find that you feel worse after using an inhaled asthma medication, check with your doctor to see if it contains sulfites.

It is estimated that 1 to 2 percent of adults and 8 percent of children have food allergies, a number that is probably higher in asthmatics. One study reported 29 percent of asthmatics as having "clinical sensitivity to food."[6] Testing for food allergies can employ various methods, including the "scratch-and-prick" technique to a food elimination diet.

There is limited evidence that a "hypoallergenic diet" may help asthmatic infants; one study reported that "90 percent of infants with allergic rhinitis and/or bronchial asthma improved on a hypoallergenic diet."[7] Hypoallergenic diets rely on "prolonged" breast-feeding with the mother avoiding cow's milk, eggs, and fish for three months. Studies on hypoallergenic diets in adults remain mixed; however, there seems to be a consensus that food allergies should be considered in asthmatics. One report from the Colorado Allergy and Asthma Center recommends that "the work-up of food allergy in asthma should be considered in patients in whom asthma is poorly controlled despite persistent use of appropriate asthma medications."[8]

Conventional Approach—Some physicians give a challenge dose of the offending drug to document a reaction. If a drug allergy is identified, an alternative medication is often prescribed. As for food allergies, most doctors will ask you to keep a food diary along with an asthma diary. Formal food allergy testing is available, but after reviewing your diaries most physicians will simply tell you to stop eating the suspected offending food.

Integrative Approach—While this method is not too different from the conventional approach, your doctor may also find a natural alternative to the offending drug. Formal food or drug testing is often indicated when there is any doubt.

Environmental Asthma

Many authorities blame the asthma epidemic on increasing levels of air pollution, especially indoor air pollution. There is little doubt that the air we breathe has become more toxic over the past thirty years. Air pollution is a leading airway irritant, and the number of hospital visits for respiratory illness increases predictably and dramatically as air quality deteriorates. This is especially true on hot, humid days or days when there are thermal inversions (which occur when a layer of cold air is trapped under a layer of warm air). While the list of asthma irritants is extensive, ozone, nitrogen dioxide, and sulfur dioxide are the greatest offenders.

Conventional and Integrative Approach—Remove the source of the air pollution, ventilate your home, and use air-conditioning on hot, humid days. Chapter 6 is devoted to cleaning the air you breathe.

Occupational or Work-Related Asthma

While I believe that work is good for you and builds character, for some asthmatics work is the cause of their trouble. Many people have occupational asthma without even knowing it. The occupational asthmatic feels fine at the start of the work week, only to have their symptoms progressively worsen over the course of the week. They often feel a little better when they go home, but their symptoms recur once they return to work the next day. Most commonly, occupational asthmatics feel best over the weekend or after a vacation, but as soon as they go back to work, their symptoms return.

The number of occupational asthma triggers is extensive and can range from wood or metal dust to chemical fumes to grains and herbs. Talk to your doctor if you have contact with any of these substances or notice that your asthma gets worse at work but better when at home.

Conventional and Integrative Approach—Identify the offending agent and remove it or avoid it. For some people, occupational asthma may be "cured" by a simple request to remove the substance. Other asthmatics may find it necessary to change careers or initiate legal action. Useful tips to help identify and remove occupational asthma triggers can be found in Chapter 6.

Exercise-Induced Asthma

People with exercise-induced asthma (EIA) typically complain of wheezing and shortness of breath after exercise. While there was once debate over whether individuals with EIA were really asthmatic, it is now generally believed that people with EIA have subclinical asthma, which will ultimately develop into chronic asthma provoked by stimuli other than exercise. It is estimated that over 70 percent of asthmatic children have EIA. Unlike allergic or infectious asthma, EIA does not result in residual airway hyperreactivity. In other words, once the EIA attack has resolved, airway reactivity returns to normal. Another difference between EIA and typical asthma is that bronchial smooth-muscle contraction does not appear to contribute to EIA. Rather, researchers suspect that the extreme temperature difference between the relatively cold, dry inhaled air and the moist, warm lung tissue causes reflex-induced lung congestion. There is, however, evidence that EIA and regular asthma may be more similar than previously thought, as one 2002 study demonstrated when it found that eosinophil levels correlated to the severity of EIA.[9]

In large part, EIA symptoms depend on the conditions under which exercise is performed. In general, the higher the ventilatory rate, the more severe the EIA. For example, EIA is more likely to occur during running rather than walking. Also, the colder and dryer the air, the more likely one will experience EIA. This is why some asthmatics have trouble with winter sports but feel fine while swimming in a heated indoor pool.

Conventional Approach—Most physicians recommend two albuterol inhalations fifteen minutes prior to exercise. If albuterol fails to control EIA symptoms, a cromolyn nasal inhaler is usually added. Cromolyn for EIA is dosed at two puffs four times a day, with an additional two puffs thirty minutes prior to exercise. See the section on exercise in Chapter 5 for tips on how to prevent EIA.

Integrative Approach—See the exercise section in Chapter 5 to learn how to avoid EIA. Chapter 7 includes information on how vitamin C can help prevent EIA.

Gastroesophageal Reflux-Associated Asthma

This is an asthma subtype not seen in many medical textbooks, however, there is an increasing body of evidence implicating gastroesophageal reflux disease (GERD) as an important player in asthma, especially asthma that is worse at night. GERD occurs when acid from the stomach finds its way up into the esophagus. Researchers suspect that this esophageal acid induces a nerve-mediated reflex that results in bronchoconstriction. An alternative theory is that this acid is aspirated into the lungs, where it causes asthmalike symptoms. Whatever the mechanism, it is estimated that 50 to 80 percent of asthmatics have GERD, although there is presently a controversy over how much asthma is caused by GERD. The interesting thing about GERD is that it doesn't always cause symptoms like heartburn. Apparently most people experience some degree of reflux, but why some individuals develop symptoms whereas others don't remains a mystery.

There are multiple studies on the relationship between GERD and asthma. One study from Iceland, published in *Chest* in 2002, examined 2,661 individuals, ranging in age from twenty to forty-eight, from three European nations. The study found that those patients who had GERD were 2.5 times more likely to have wheezing and almost 3 times more likely to have shortness of breath at night, when compared to people who did not have GERD. The authors concluded that "the occurrence of [GERD] after bedtime is strongly associated with both asthma and respiratory symptoms."[10] Another study examined fifty-two children with various respiratory symptoms and found that in 42.2 percent of these patients, GERD was the cause of their chronic respiratory symptoms.[11] A group of Italian researchers summed up the link between GERD and asthma, writing that "in patients with asthma, nocturnal [GERD] has been associated with triggering and worsening bronchoconstriction. There are data to suggest that the prevalence of [GERD] is higher in patients with asthma than in the general population and that [GERD] is directly associated with asthma severity."[12]

Even more remarkable, there is a substantial body of evidence demonstrating that some asthmatics will have their asthma "cured" following anti-reflux therapy. One French study followed forty-four patients with severe asthma who had their GERD treated surgically. The authors reported that 25 percent of these patients experienced "total cure" of their asthma and another 16 percent experienced "marked improvement."[13] Another study, which examined 324 patients who had GERD-related asthma, chest pain, cough, and hoarseness, found that 94 percent reported improved symptoms and 48 percent had their symptoms resolve following surgery.[14] Children may have more to gain from reflux surgery, considering one study of 132 children and adults found that 78.6 percent of the children had their respiratory symptoms disappear after surgery compared to 36 percent of adults.[15]

If you have severe asthma with GERD, surgery is an option you may want to investigate. Further studies on medical versus surgical management of GERD in asthmatics are underway. How much GERD actually contributes to asthma will probably remain a subject of debate for some time; however, if you find your asthma symptoms are particularly worse at night, consider the possibility that GERD is playing a role. A trial of anti-reflux therapy may be warranted, so talk to your healthcare provider about your concerns and treatment options.

ASTHMA CLASSIFICATIONS REVISITED

In the real world, most people share features of several different types of asthma. For instance, someone could have seasonal allergic asthma and also be sensitive to cooking smells. Further complicating matters is that sensitivities can change over time and what is troublesome for a particular asthmatic today may not bother him or her two years later. If any generalizations can be made, it is that childhood asthma tends to be allergic, whereas adult-onset asthma is usually mixed or idiosyncratic. Despite these limitations, such classifications are useful for talking about asthma and, as will become more apparent in the following chapters, for treating and preventing asthma. In the next chapter, you'll learn ways to help determine what type of asthmatic you are. This is important because if you know what triggers your symptoms, you can learn to control those triggers, a vital step toward living a symptom-free life without medications.

DIAGNOSING ASTHMA

Diagnosing asthma can be tricky simply because most asthmatics only have occasional symptoms. For most people, asthma tends to come and go with symptom-free periods that can last for days or months. If you see your doctor when you're not having symptoms, it may be difficult to establish the diagnosis. Adding to this difficulty is that, even among physicians, there is controversy over how to define asthma. Despite this, most physicians will use personal history followed by a variety of clinical and laboratory tests to make the diagnosis.

Most doctors can make a presumptive diagnosis of asthma after listening to your complaints and doing a physical exam. To establish a diagnosis, however, formal pulmonary testing is needed. The "gold standard" for measuring lung function is called the Pulmonary Function Test (PFT). During the PFT, a person blows into a machine that measures a variety of lung volumes. Sometimes a less complicated machine called a spirometer is used to make these measurements. For the asthmatic, the most important measurements are the Forced Expiratory Volume (FEV) and Forced Expiratory Volume in One Second (FEV_1).

FEV is the volume of air you can force out from your lungs. FEV is measured by having you take the deepest breath possible, then blowing all the air out into the PFT machine. FEV_1 is the amount of air you can blow out in one second after taking the deepest breath possible. By measuring FEV and FEV_1, we can determine how well your lungs work. If FEV and FEV_1 are measured during as asthma attack, the severity of the attack can be accurately determined.

Normal FEV and FEV_1 values vary from person to person and depend in part on age and height. As we age, there is a normal reduction in lung function that is reflected by a lower FEV and FEV_1. Conversely, the taller you are, the bigger your lungs tend to be, which can increase your FEV and FEV_1. FEV and FEV_1 measurements are expressed as a percentage of predicted normal. Given the wide fluctuations in asthma, FEV and FEV_1 can range from perfectly normal to less than 10 percent of predicted normal. In fact, most asthmatics have normal FEV and FEV_1 except when they have an attack.

Asthma symptoms are usually perceived when FEV drops below 50 percent of predicted normal or the RV doubles. RV, or residual volume, is another lung measure representing the amount of air left in the lungs after completely exhaling. As mentioned earlier, asthma has more to do with not getting air out of the lungs than getting air in, and during an attack air can be trapped in the lungs. During a severe attack, RV can increase to four times normal.

While FEV and FEV_1 are useful measures of lung function, these measurements alone cannot definitively establish a diagnosis of asthma. First of all, the measurements must be taken during an attack. Second, even if FEV and FEV_1 are abnormal, this finding can be caused by another medical condition, such as emphysema or chronic bronchitis. In order to nail a diagnosis of asthma, we have to demonstrate hyperreactivity and reversibility, in addition to recording abnormal FEV and FEV_1.

Asthmatic airways are overly sensitive, or hyperreactive, which can lead to reversible bronchoconstriction. We test for hyperreactivity by measuring the reduction in FEV and FEV_1 after inhalation of a known bronchoconstrictor, such as methacholine, histamine, or cold air. Most people will experience mild airway narrowing when exposed to these stimuli; however, asthmatics have an exaggerated response that results in significantly abnormal FEV and FEV_1.

Once we have established that the lungs are hyperreactive, we can then test for reversibility by giving the patient a bronchodilator and remeasuring FEV_1. An increase in FEV_1 of 15 percent or more after bronchodilator inhalation is considered a positive test for reversible bronchoconstriction. Hence, a definitive diagnosis of asthma can only be made with an appropriate clinical history coupled with PFT-documented airway hyperreactivity and reversible bronchoconstriction.

Many doctors feel comfortable diagnosing asthma on clinical grounds alone, with PFT reserved for those cases where the diagnosis is in question. I believe that most people with wheezing should have a PFT as well as a bronchoconstrictor challenge. These tests are recommended not only to measure asthma severity but also to establish a definitive diagnosis, excluding the possibility of misdiagnosis.

WHY YOU SHOULD GET A SECOND OPINION AND INSIST ON THE HIGHEST STANDARD

Should you be concerned about receiving the wrong diagnosis? Presented with the classic symptoms, most doctors are correct when they make a diagnosis of asthma. Nobody is perfect, however, and when a doctor makes a mistake in diagnosing asthma, the consequences can be severe. This is why it is always wise to get a second opinion. You may learn that your asthma is not as severe as first suspected or discover that you don't even have asthma.

Warning signs that may mean misdiagnosis include a new diagnosis of asthma over age forty or symptoms that fail to get better with treatment. Most people with asthma are diagnosed prior to age forty and any new diagnosis after age forty should be held suspect. Suspicion is also warranted for the patient who does not respond to standard therapy. For a physician, this means one of five things:

- You've made the wrong diagnosis.
- You've made the right diagnosis, but the patient has severe disease.
- You've made the right diagnosis, but chosen the wrong medicine.
- You've made the right diagnosis, but the primary trigger has not been removed (for example, a cat).
- You've made the right diagnosis, but the patient is not following your directions.

A healthy dose of skepticism never hurt and will keep your doctor on his or her toes. Remember, it's your life, not the doctor's, and you have the most to lose in all of this. You and your doctor should also be aware that there are several medical conditions that can masquerade as asthma and may need to be eliminated as possibilities.

Because GERD is such a common condition and a known asthma trigger, talk to your doctor about being tested for GERD, especially if you have symptoms like heartburn. Many asthmatics report improved symptoms once their GERD is treated.

Dysfunctional breathing goes by many names, including behavioral breathlessness and hyperventilation syndrome. No matter what you call it, dysfunctional breathing adds up to a breathing disorder characterized by hyperventilation. Not only does dysfunctional breathing contribute to asthma, but it can be mistaken for asthma and lead to a misdiagnosis. It is suspected that therapies like Buteyko Breathing and yoga are so helpful to asthmatics because they train people how to breathe properly (to learn more about breathing therapy for asthma, see Chapter 9). Given how common dysfunctional breathing is among asthmatics, ask your doctor if this disorder may be contributing to your symptoms.

Asthmalike symptoms can also be caused by chronic bronchitis. Bronchitis is an inflammation of the large airways and is usually caused by infection. Like GERD, treating the bronchitis may cure the "asthma." Another lung disorder that can cause asthmalike symptoms is allergic bronchopulmonary aspergillosis, a fungal infection of the lung. People with heart failure can have their symptoms confused with asthma, because heart failure can cause pulmonary edema that results in wheezing and shortness of breath. Known as "cardiac asthma," these symptoms disappear once the heart problem is treated.

Bronchiectasis is an uncommon medical condition in which the lung's airways become dilated and stiff, resulting in asthmalike symptoms. The glottis, which helps keep food you swallow from entering your lungs, can also cause airway obstruction if it is not working properly. Other rare conditions that can cause airway problems are tumors, foreign bodies (for example, accidentally swallowed objects), vocal cord dysfunction, and laryngeal (voice box) edema.

When visiting your doctor, suggest the possibility that another medical condition is causing your symptoms. Chances are, if your doctor thinks you have asthma, you probably have asthma; however, by mentioning these possibilities, you get your doctor to think more broadly about your condition and, if indicated, order the necessary tests.

OK, YOU HAVE ASTHMA—WHAT'S NEXT?

So, you got a second opinion and, yes, you have asthma. What's next? First, let your doctor help you get your symptoms under control. Stabilizing your asthma is important not only because you'll feel better physically and emotionally, but also so you can eventually rid yourself of asthma. Right now, however, I suggest you trust your doctor. Your physician knows what is needed to stabilize your asthma and put control back in your hands.

You may prefer not to use drugs, but if your doctor believes medication is best for right now, do as your doctor says. There are many people in this world who would not be alive today had it not been for asthma medicine. Medications, when appropriately prescribed, help far more people than they hurt. Later, once your symptoms have calmed down and you've learned what aggravates your asthma, then you and your physician can look at ways to control your asthma rather than having asthma control you.

The next thing you need to do is take a deep breath and relax. Asthma can be treated and controlled—even beat. View your asthma as a wake-up call that the body is not indestructible, that your body needs care and attention. After I accepted my diagnosis, my world changed and I started to pay attention to how I treated my body. These changes did not come overnight but evolved over several years, until one day I said, "Hey, this is bull—I control my life, my asthma doesn't." Once I took control, my life turned around. Since then, I have been fundamentally drug-free, having gone from seven medications to the occasional one. At the age of forty-two, I can honestly say I'm in great shape. My life changed because I have asthma—it changed for the better. Now that you have asthma, your life can also change for the better.

chapter 3

What Type of Asthmatic Are You?

KNOW THYSELF—THE WORDS RING TRUE for every part of life, but they are especially important for the asthmatic. Learning about asthma and knowing what type of asthmatic you are not only will save your life (which, as we learned, is really the least of your problems), but also will enable you to live the life you deserve. Experts share the sentiment that knowing about asthma is a powerful weapon against the disease. This belief is echoed in a report from Northwestern Health Sciences University, which concluded that "the increased sense of control and knowledge about the asthmatic condition is likely to have resulted in anxiety reduction, contributed to proper medication use, and thus may also explain some of the observed improvements in [asthma] outcome."[1] Bottom line: The more you know about asthma, the better you can control asthma.

There are three basic, related questions we will answer in this chapter:

- How severe is your asthma?
- How well controlled is your asthma?
- What triggers your asthma?

The purpose of this book is to get you medication-free or dramatically reduce the number of medications you use. In this chapter, I describe the types of asthmatics who should never reduce their medication without a physician's guidance. If you're one of these asthmatics, don't despair. Most of this book is about how to change your life and environment so that your asthma no longer becomes an issue. This advice applies to everyone, from the most stable, mild asthmatic to the bed-bound, steroid-dependent asthmatic. If you have severe asthma, don't concentrate on how many medications you're taking. Instead, concentrate on changing your environment and how you live, and, before you know it, you and your doctor will be cutting back on your medicine.

HOW SEVERE IS YOUR ASTHMA?

While it may be true that under the right circumstances any asthmatic can have a severe attack, most asthmatics have relatively consistent symptoms. One asthma attack usually doesn't vary much from the last and, as we learned in Chapter 1, many asthmatics improve over time. There are several ways to gauge the severity of your asthma. The first and easiest way is to ask your doctor. Because asthma is an exceptionally common condition, many doctors have significant experience treating it and are thereby capable of determining its severity.

Peak Flow Readings

You can personally estimate the severity of an attack, and hence the severity of your asthma, by using a peak flow meter. Asthma attacks are graded from mild to moderate to severe, and severity is calculated by comparing Predicted Peak Flow (PPF) or Best Peak Flow (BPF) to current peak flow. Keep in mind that peak flow readings are effort dependent, so always give your best shot or else the reading may not be accurate. If you hold back on how hard you blow or don't use proper technique, you can make a mild attack seem, at least according to the peak flow meter, like a severe attack. You may think no harm is done, but imagine the psychological impact on the mild asthmatic whose peak flow meter is telling them it's time to call 911. So, whenever you whip out your peak flow meter, make sure you give it your best shot.

It's always a good idea to have your peak flow technique observed by a healthcare professional to make sure you're using the meter correctly. Also, when visiting your doctor, always bring your asthma journal with peak flow recordings. Allowing your physician to see the numbers, rather than just telling him or her about the numbers, is absolutely critical to helping your physician make informed decisions.

Every asthmatic should know his or her Best Peak Flow (BPF), the highest peak flow you can achieve when your asthma is well controlled. BPF is different from Predicted Peak Flow (PPF), an estimate of what your peak flow should be given your sex, age, and height (see Tables 3.1 and 3.2 on

A Little Doctor's Office in Your Pocket

A peak flow meter is like a little doctor's office you can carry in your pocket that measures how much air you can exhale from your lungs. For an asthmatic, this measurement depends on whether or not you're having symptoms. Peak flow drops during an asthma attack and rises to normal once the attack is over. Peak flow meters are small, inexpensive, and your doctor may have already given you a free one. You should also keep an asthma journal (discussed further in Chapter 3), a diary that will help you keep track of your peak flow measurements and monitor your asthma symptoms. Even more important, your asthma journal is going to help you get rid of your asthma. One of the best ways to determine the severity of an asthma attack is to measure your peak flow and compare this reading to your Best Peak Flow (BPF).

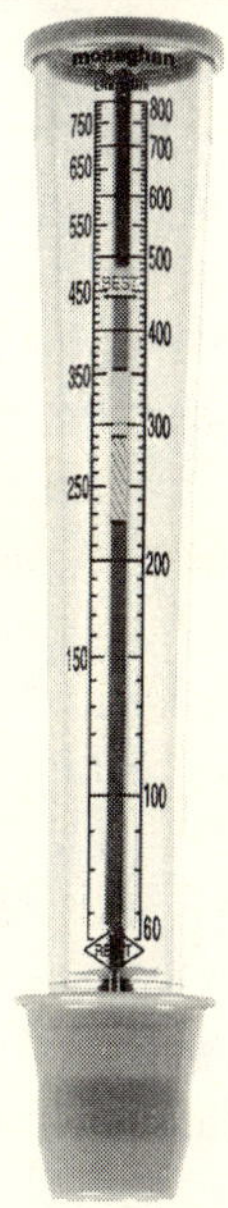

Figure 3.1. TruZone Peak Flow Meter showing representative ColorZone regions, indicated by the shaded central core. ColorZone regions are applied using transparent ColorZone tape and vary between individuals.

The peak flow meter has two ends, one end you blow into and one end through which the blown air escapes. Traveling between the two ends, the air moves a spring-loaded piston attached to an indicator that records your peak flow in liters per minute (L/min). Here's how to use a peak flow meter:

1. Zero your peak flow meter by moving the indicator to the zero position.
2. While standing, take as deep a breath as you can, then hold this breath while wrapping your lips tightly around the peak flow mouthpiece.
3. Try to blow all the air out as hard and fast as you can into the peak flow meter while keeping a tight seal between your lips and the mouthpiece.
4. Record the peak flow in your asthma journal with the date, time, and circumstances, then zero the peak flow meter.
5. Repeat this procedure two more times and record each reading. If you cough or don't achieve a good seal with the mouthpiece, don't record the result.

page 51). For instance, the PPF for a twenty-year-old, seventy-inch-tall male is 649 liters a minute. The reason why BPF is the preferred measure for asthmatics is that many people, even those without asthma, have a BPF that is significantly higher or lower than their PPF. BPF tells you how you are doing in relation to your normal readings, not to the rest of the population.

Comparing present peak flow to BPF is a more accurate reflection of how well or poorly your asthma is doing. To determine your BPF, take two or three peak flow readings daily when your asthma is stable. Record these peak flows after you wake up and in the early afternoon between noon and 2 P.M. You should also record your peak flow before and after using a short-acting beta-agonist like albuterol. After you have accumulated two to three weeks of readings, ask your physician to review the numbers to determine your Best Peak Flow. Your BPF will usually be your highest peak flow reading. If you've just returned from the closet and are dusting off your old peak flow meter, don't be surprised if your BPF is lower than several years ago, as peak flow naturally declines with age. Hence, most authorities recommend that you determine your BPF every six months.

We are interested in comparing your most recent BPF to your peak flow during an asthma attack. You can measure the severity of an asthma attack by taking a peak flow reading during the attack and calculating the percentage change from BPF. Let's calculate a sample percentage change in peak flow following the simple formula, Severity of asthma attack equals current peak flow divided by Best Peak Flow. If your BPF is 700 L/min and you're now blowing 550 L/min, how bad is this attack? Divide current peak flow by BPF: 550/700 = 0.79 (79 percent). During this attack, your current peak flow represents 79 percent of your BPF. You are having a mild asthma attack.

Like a traffic light, asthma severity is divided into green, yellow, and red zones, otherwise known as the PEF (Peak Expiratory Flow) Zone system:

- **Green Zone**—If your peak flow is greater than 80 percent of your BPF, your asthma is well controlled; if you take any medications, take them as usual.
- **Yellow Zone**—If your peak flow is 50 to 80 percent of BPF, you are having a mild to moderate asthma attack and should take a short-acting beta2-agonist; ask your doctor if you need to change your daily medication regimen.

Table 3.1: Predicted Peak Flow for Adult Men
(Liters/Minute)

AGE	HEIGHT 60 inches	65 inches	70 inches	75 inches
20	554	602	649	693
25	543	590	636	679
30	532	577	622	664
35	521	565	609	651
40	509	552	596	636
45	498	540	583	622
50	486	527	569	607
55	475	515	556	593
60	463	502	542	578
65	452	490	529	564
70	440	477	515	550

Table 3.2: Predicted Peak Flow for Adult Women
(Liters/Minute)

AGE	HEIGHT 55 inches	60 inches	65 inches	70 inches
20	390	423	460	496
25	385	418	454	490
30	380	413	448	483
35	375	408	442	476
40	370	402	436	470
45	365	397	430	464
50	360	391	424	457
55	355	386	418	451
60	350	380	412	445
65	345	375	406	439
70	340	369	400	432

- **Red Zone**—If your peak flow is less than 50 percent of BPF, you are having a severe asthma attack and, in addition to taking a short-acting beta2-agonist, you should call your doctor or go to the nearest emergency room.

After inhaling a beta-agonist, you should ideally see a 20 percent increase in peak flow. For further information on how to manage an acute asthma attack, talk to your physician. Table 3.3 on page 53 can be used to make calculating your percent change in peak flow easy. For instance, if your BPF is 500 and you are now blowing 350, you are within 60 to 80 percent of your BPF and are in the yellow zone. If, however, you are blowing 240, your current peak flow is less than 60 percent of your BPF and you are in the red zone.

Most physicians will recommend that you take routine daily peak flow measurements even when you're feeling well. Multiple peak flow measurements track baseline lung function and can detect airway narrowing hours to days before an attack, allowing for early intervention prior to symptom development. Talk to your healthcare professional about how your peak flow meter can detect an attack before symptoms occur.

There are exceptions to every rule, but in most cases measuring your peak flow is an excellent way to follow the severity of your asthma. The only major problem with peak flow is that the reading you get after you blow into your meter depends in large part on how hard you blow; that is, peak flow measurements are effort dependent. This is why when you measure peak flow, remember to give it your best shot. To get the most accurate reading, it's also important to take three peak flow measurements in a row and, even more important, to know how to use a peak flow meter.

Other Signs of Asthma Severity

While peak flow readings give you an idea of the severity of an asthma attack, they don't tell the whole story. To know how severe your asthma is, we have to examine your history because past asthma behavior is often predictive of future asthma behavior. If the majority of your attacks are mild, and you know that over the past ten years one attack never varied much from the next, we can safely say you have mild asthma. The same logic holds for moderate and severe asthma. While most asthmatics have predictable symptoms, the rare subtype brittle asthma is characterized by severe, unpredictable attacks that can occur without warning. If you've

Table 3.3: Easy Reference Chart for Calculating Percent Change in Peak Flow

Your Best Peak Flow (L/min)	Percentage of your BPF		Your Best Peak Flow (L/min)	Percentage of your BPF	
	80%	60%		80%	60%
750	600	450	475	380	285
725	580	435	450	360	270
700	560	420	425	340	255
675	540	405	400	320	240
650	520	390	375	300	225
625	500	375	350	280	210
600	480	360	325	260	195
575	460	345	300	240	180
550	440	330	275	220	165
525	420	315	250	200	150
500	400	300	225	180	135

ever been diagnosed with brittle or severe asthma, always work with your doctor when changing your medication regimen.

A sure sign of severe asthma is a history of intubation, being put on a ventilator with a tube down your throat to help you breathe. In my mind, intubation immediately puts you in the severe category no matter how well controlled you are today. You may be feeling great right now, but a history of intubation means there's a significant risk of a severe attack. So, if you were ever intubated (or nearly intubated), it is especially important that you work closely with a doctor to get your asthma under control.

Another way to appreciate asthma severity involves the number and types of medications you take. If you use only one or two medications, like albuterol and an inhaled steroid, chances are your asthma is mild. If, however, you require four to ten medications, this indicates moderate to severe asthma. Most doctors would also agree that necessary oral steroid use is a warning sign of moderate to severe asthma, with chronic oral steroid use or "steroid dependency" indicative of severe asthma.

A history of hospitalization also figures into the asthma severity equation. Having been hospitalized for asthma puts you in the moderate to severe category. Emergency-room visits are more difficult to assess. When I see someone who has been in the emergency room but never admitted to the hospital, it means either they have mild to severe asthma that is poorly controlled or they have mild to severe asthma that responded well to the usual emergency room treatments. In other words, the number of emergency-room visits doesn't tell a whole lot about severity, but it is a good predictor of overall asthma control. When evaluating asthma severity, most doctors rely on prior history, medication use, and hospitalization and/or intubation history.

If you find that you fall into the severe or brittle asthma category, don't give up. Having severe asthma only means you have to move slower and work more closely with your doctor. Most of this book is devoted to removing asthma triggers and strengthening your body and immune system so they can defend your lungs against the toxic rigors of life. The advice given here is intended for everyone, no matter how mild or severe his or her asthma. The degree of asthma severity will only impact these recommendations by altering how quickly the necessary lifestyle and medication changes can and should be made. Obviously, we can be more aggressive with a mild, stable asthmatic on one or two medications than with a brittle asthmatic who has just been discharged from the hospital and takes ten different medications. No matter what your situation, I recommend you form an alliance with an understanding and trusted doctor who can safely guide you through these changes.

HOW WELL CONTROLLED ARE YOU?

The question of control in many ways ties into the severity of your asthma. Control, however, does not necessarily translate into severity, as you can have a severe asthmatic with wonderful control and a mild asthmatic with horrible control. When I ask a patient how well their asthma is controlled, I'm actually asking several questions. I first want to know how often they use their medicine, especially their albuterol inhaler. Albuterol is normally used for "rescue therapy," to stop an acute asthma attack, or prophylactically, such as prior to exercise to prevent exercise-induced asthma. An asthmatic with excellent control rarely, if ever, uses their albuterol inhaler. Asthmatics who need their albuterol inhaler daily are poorly controlled no matter how severe or mild their asthma may be.

Like severity, the control question also involves hospital and emergency-room visits. Most asthmatics never see the inside of an emergency room, while some asthmatics are in the emergency room weekly. If you've been in the hospital or emergency room even once over the past two years, I would be concerned about how well controlled you are.

Steroid use is sometimes an indication of poor or difficult control. Some people with mild, normally well-controlled asthma occasionally need a short course of steroids to help them over a rough spot, such as after a cold. At the other end of the spectrum is the severe, steroid-dependent asthmatic who is well controlled as long as he or she keeps taking steroids. Like emergency-room visits that don't necessarily correlate to asthma severity, steroid use when examined alone doesn't offer much information about how well controlled an asthmatic is.

When evaluating asthma stability, most physicians will look at medication use as well as hospital and emergency-room visits. If you have unstable asthma, I suggest you throw yourself at the mercy of the medical profession to stabilize your asthma. Once your asthma is stable, then you and your doctor can talk about cutting back on medications.

WHAT TRIGGERS YOUR ASTHMA?

Without a doubt, the most important question is "What triggers your asthma?" Like those cute battery commercials on TV, what sets off your "asthma bunny" and keeps it going and going? If you can find the culprit and remove it from your environment, chances are you will be bothered by asthma no more. Sounds great, doesn't it? I hope that after reading this book, some of you will quickly find that magic trigger and rid yourself of asthma. Most of you, however, will have to do some detective work. There will be some trial and error, but if you are patient and methodical, you will discover what makes your asthma tick and conquer it.

You probably know a lot about your asthma already, and I'm sure most of you can name five to ten things that contribute to your attacks. After reading Chapter 2, you probably even know what type of asthmatic you tend to be and realize that your asthma often shares the features of several different subtypes. While these asthma subtypes are somewhat artificial, they make us better asthma detectives. For those of you who think you have idiopathic asthma, after digging a little deeper we'll probably find at least a couple of things that trigger your asthma. The most important task of an asthma detective is to ask five basic questions each time you have an attack:

- Where am I?

- What am I doing?
- What is around me?
- Do I know what set off this attack?
- How severe is this attack?

After you answer these questions, take out your asthma journal and record the answers, along with the date and time of the attack. Everyone has their own method of keeping an asthma diary, but the following information is standard and will help you and your physician immensely in determining what gets your asthma hopping.

- Date: Date attack started.
- Time: Time you first noticed symptoms.
- Location: Where you were at the beginning of the attack.
- Circumstances: What you were doing when the attack started.
- Trigger: What you know or suspect triggered the attack. If it is a suspicion, put a "?" next to the trigger.
- Severity: How severe you believe the attack is before measuring peak flow. Use a mild-moderate-severe scale.
- Peak Flow During Attack: Actual peak flow during the attack. Remember to take and record three readings.
- Treatment/Interventions: How you attempted to abort the attack. For example, record what type and how much medicine you used, or what you did (for instance, just relax, breathing exercise) in an attempt to relieve your symptoms.
- Time to Resolution: How long it took to feel that the attack was over after the intervention.
- Efficacy: Did the intervention(s) work? Yes, no, or maybe.
- Duration of Attack: How long the attack lasted, from the time you first noticed symptoms to the time you believed the attack was over.
- Peak Flow After Intervention: Peak flow reading at the time you believed the attack was over. Once again, take and record three readings.

Keeping an asthma diary may seem like a pain; however, not only will your diary help you figure out what triggers your asthma, but the simple act of keeping an asthma diary may help your lung function. In one randomized trial, asthmatics who recorded stressful life events in a journal increased their FEV_1 from 63.9 L at the beginning of the trial to 76.3 L after sixteen weeks; on the other hand, the control group started with a FEV_1 of 64.0 L and ended with a FEV_1 of only 65.3 L.

I hope that by recording this data you begin to recognize patterns. You may find that your asthma tends to be worse when in a certain room or performing a particular activity. Share your diary with your healthcare professional and a trusted friend or two, because you never know what a fresh eye may discover.

Interrogation Time

OK, I'm turning on the bright lights and oiling up the thumbscrews, because it's time to ask some hard questions and discover what triggers your asthma. Before we begin, take a moment to write down five to ten things you know trigger an attack. For instance, one day my wife bought some new perfume. The only problem was that the perfume immediately triggered my asthma. Needless to say, that brand of perfume will never find its way into my home again. I want you to have this same take-no-prisoners approach to your asthma triggers. If it's on your list, it should be in the trash! This technique is called "source control" (which we will learn in Chapter 6) and is without a doubt the most effective way to treat asthma. As you answer the questions that follow, you'll find that some asthma triggers are easy to identify and remove, whereas others require some investigation and hard decisions. The most important thing you can do right now is trash those triggers you know about and faithfully note all possible triggers in your asthma diary. What follows is a list of questions that, while far from exhaustive, offers an excellent starting point to get you thinking about your asthma and what sets it off.

Where Do You Live? What Do You Do?

- *Do you live in the city, country, or suburbs?* Cockroaches are notorious asthma triggers and city folk shouldn't underestimate the tenacity of a cockroach or overestimate the cleanliness of their building. Adding to their troubles, urban asthmatics often have outdoor air pollution to contend with. For those in the country, agriculture and pollen are frequent troublemakers. Suburban dwellers have to contend with all three: air pollution, agriculture, and pollen. Everyone, no matter where they live, should investigate sources of indoor and outdoor air pollution, the focus of Chapter 6.

- *Do you live in a single-family home?* Well, at least you don't have to worry about your neighbor being a cockroach breeder. You or your neighbor may, however, have a garden acting as a pollen factory. Read Chapter 6 to learn how to asthma-proof your home.
- *Do you live in an apartment or condominium?* Time to think about the cleanliness of your neighbor. Perhaps it's his dog that spreads dander throughout the building. Keeping your apartment or condo meticulously clean and free of dust goes a long way in helping your asthma.
- *Do you have a garden?* Two words: fungus and pollen. If your asthma is worse in your garden, you don't have to dig deeply to know what's causing the problem. All that moist soil and those pretty flowers spew forth all sorts of fungi and pollen just waiting to land in a cozy warm place like your airways. Rather than paving your yard with asphalt, consider a Japanese rock garden or growing non-pollinating, asthma-friendly plants. If you can't live without flowers, keep your windows facing the garden closed, especially during allergy season.
- *What type of work do you do?* Occupational asthma is common and the list of triggers is almost endless. Typically with work-related asthma, the asthma is worse at work but gets a little better at home and a lot better on vacation, only to worsen upon returning to work. As it raises the possibility of litigation, work-related asthma is a touchy subject for employees and employers. Nevertheless, if you suspect your workplace is causing your symptoms, talk to your doctor and start listing the materials you work with. The best-case scenario is you'll find what's triggering your asthma and have it removed without a hassle. The worst-case scenario could involve attorneys and/or changing jobs, even careers.
- *What are your hobbies?* Some people use airplane glue to build models while others smoke their own meats. Ask yourself if your asthma feels better or worse while enjoying your hobby.

What Time of Day, Week, or Year Is Your Asthma Worse?

- *Is your asthma worse during a certain time of the year?* If your symptoms are worse during the spring or fall, chances are you have seasonal allergies triggering your asthma. Seasonal allergies boil down to an air-quality problem, so the recommendations found in Chapter 6 work equally well for allergies. Besides cleaning the air you breathe, consider a non-sedating antihistamine or a natural remedy like vitamin C. If your symptoms are worse during the winter, you're probably sensitive to cold air and may need to breathe through a face mask that warms and humidifies the air before it reaches your lungs.

- *Is your asthma worse during the morning or at night?* Bedtime symptoms may indicate a dust-mite allergy or gastroesophageal reflux disease (GERD). If you notice that your asthma acts up during a certain time of day, note where you are and what you're doing.
- *Does your asthma improve over the weekend?* If your asthma gets better over the weekend, when away from work, you may have occupational asthma. This can be caused by something like a coworker's cologne or the materials you work with. For example, some asthmatics are sensitive to wood dust, a big problem if you're in construction.
- *Does your asthma get better or disappear while you're on vacation?* An asthma-free vacation means that something in your home, workplace, or local environment is triggering your asthma. In fact, an asthma-free vacation is strong evidence that something identifiable is responsible for your symptoms. Your mission is to identify this trigger and remove it from your environment.

Where Is Your Asthma Worse?

- *Is your asthma worse at home?* Some people have asthma only at home. If this applies to you, start snooping around your house, room by room, to see where your asthma is worse. Performing a complete home search for asthma triggers is very important and is the focus of Chapter 6, where you will learn that the home is packed with asthma precipitators. You will also learn several quick and easy ways to make your home more asthma friendly.
- *Is your asthma worse in the bedroom?* Dust mites are known to cause asthma in sensitized individuals and are found in the best bedrooms of America.
- *Is your asthma worse in the kitchen?* Cooking creates products of com-

bustion that, when inhaled, deliver a major oxidative stress to the lungs. The kitchen is also home to cooking and food smells that can drive some asthmatics nuts! See Chapter 6 for how to create an asthma-safe kitchen.

- *Is your asthma worse in the bathroom?* The bathroom is another hot spot for asthma triggers, with its steady supply of scented soaps, perfumes, cleaning agents, and even mold, all of which can trigger an asthma attack.
- *Is your asthma worse in the garage?* Besides auto fumes, you'd be surprised by what people keep in their garage. Pesticides, chemicals, and cleaning agents can all cause asthma trouble. Properly dispose of those chemicals and cleaners you don't use and see Chapter 6 for more information on how to eliminate asthma-provoking noxious fumes.
- *Is your asthma worse in the living room?* Just when you thought there was an asthma-safe room in the house, I have to tell you that the living room is another potential trouble spot. Living rooms are often brimming with fluffy furniture, carpeting, and drapery that can act as pollen and allergen traps, waiting to release their asthma-triggering nectar into the air.
- *Is your asthma worse in the dining room?* Given its proximity to the kitchen, the dining room is often a victim of circumstance, with many of the same asthma triggers that are found in the kitchen.
- *Is your asthma worse in your child's room?* Kids bring all sorts of stuff home, including their aversion to tidiness. Besides being a favorite location for authorized and unauthorized pets, your child's room probably has dust balls, as well as dirt, tracked in from outside, all potential asthma triggers. Keep the kid's room just as clean as the rest of your home.
- *Is your asthma worse in the laundry room?* The laundry room—a bane of my own asthma—contains fabric softeners and scented laundry detergents that can aggravate asthma. Chapter 6 will help you clean up your laundry room.
- *Do you have any indoor plants?* Plants release pollen and sit in damp soil that is a breeding ground for mold, a known asthma irritant.
- *Is your asthma worse or better when you're at someone else's house?* If your asthma is worse at a friend's house, think about what they have

that you don't. Do they have a pet? Do they smoke? Is it your friend's perfume or cologne? If your asthma is better at a friend's house, think of what you have that your friend doesn't. This may offer clues to what is triggering your asthma.

- *Is your asthma worse in the car?* Car exhaust is a potent cause of oxidative stress known to trigger asthma. Do you leave the car's vents open when in traffic, thereby allowing exhaust fumes into your car? Is the problem an exhaust system that is leaking fumes into your car? Have your car's exhaust system checked and, when in traffic, keep the vents closed. In hot weather, close your windows and use the air-conditioning.

Do People Trigger Your Asthma?

- *Is your asthma worse when around a certain person like a boss, coworker, friend, or family member?* Sorry, asthma is no excuse to avoid your boss; however, it could be her perfume or his aftershave that's setting off your symptoms. Be suspicious of common items like grooming products, which are often overlooked as sources of asthma trouble.
- *Is your asthma worse around your wife, husband, or significant other?* You probably would not have married that person if their presence triggered an asthma attack, so whatever is giving you trouble is probably something new. Ask them about new perfumes or colognes, soaps, laundry detergents, or makeup.
- *Is your asthma worse around your children?* Before you know it, children grow up and start using adult grooming products. If suddenly your asthma acts up when your kid is around, it's time to ask some questions.
- *Is your asthma worse around a pet?* Pets and asthma usually don't mix. We'll talk more about pets in Chapter 6, but for now think critically about keeping your pet.

What Are You Eating? What Medications Are You Taking?

- *Are your symptoms worse after you eat?* Food allergies frequently contribute to asthma. Do you feel discomfort after breakfast, lunch, or dinner? If so, keep a food diary with your asthma diary to see if there is an association between what you eat and your symptoms. Share this information with your doctor, who can test for specific food allergies.
- *What medications are you taking?* Carefully review your prescription and

over-the-counter medications with your doctor. Many medicines contain preservatives or food dyes that are notorious asthma aggravators. Also, carefully examine the ingredients of natural remedies (vitamins, minerals, herbs), which can occasionally surprise you with asthma-triggering preservatives or fillers.

What Are Your Daily Activities?

- *Is your asthma worse in the shower?* Scented soaps and shampoos can cause asthma trouble. The shower is also a favorite spot for mold, so keep your shower and bathroom free of mildew.
- *Is your asthma worse after exercise?* Exercise-induced asthma (EIA) is exceptionally common and easy to treat. See Chapter 5 on how to treat and avoid EIA.
- *Is your asthma worse at night when in bed?* This could be due to those pesky dust mites. Or you may not even have asthma but gastroesophageal reflux disease (GERD), which can mimic asthma's symptoms.
- *Does vacuuming make your asthma worse?* Carpets trap all sorts of nasty stuff like cat dander, pollen, and dust. This is why carpets, especially wall-to-wall carpeting, are taboo for asthmatics.
- *Does making the bed trigger your asthma?* If making the bed aggravates your asthma, this almost certainly means you're sensitive to dust mites.
- *Does cleaning furniture make your asthma worse?* Glass and furniture cleaners are packed with chemicals that can provoke an attack. If your asthma acts up while polishing glass or furniture, try switching cleaners or, if you can stand it, have someone clean for you.

What Are Your Medical Conditions?

- *Do you have gastroesophageal reflux disease (GERD) or heartburn?* The association between GERD and asthma is well established. We know that GERD can not only make asthma symptoms worse, but can also masquerade as asthma and lead to a misdiagnosis. GERD-related asthma is usually worse at night when the individual lies down to sleep. Remember, you don't need heartburn to have GERD, so speak to your doctor about the possibility of GERD contributing to your symptoms.
- *Do you have allergies or postnasal drip?* Seasonal allergies frequently trig-

ger asthma attacks, and there are many asthmatics who gain considerable relief by avoiding allergens, taking an antihistamine, or using a natural remedy. Postnasal drip can cause a chronic cough that may be mistaken for cough-variant asthma. Ask your healthcare professional how to treat your allergies or postnasal drip.

- *Do you have heart problems, high cholesterol, or a history of heart attack?* When the heart doesn't pump well, the lungs can fill with fluid, causing shortness of breath and wheezing, a condition known as "cardiac asthma" or congestive heart failure (CHF). Since most people don't develop heart trouble until they're fifty or sixty, if you receive a diagnosis of asthma before the age of fifty and don't have a history of heart disease, you probably can't blame your heart. Conversely, any individual who receives a new diagnosis of asthma after age fifty should have their heart checked.
- *Do you smoke or have a history of smoking?* Smoking is one of the most destructive things you can do to your body, setting you up for heart disease, asthma, and emphysema. Emphysema and asthma have similar symptoms and, like heart disease, emphysema usually doesn't appear until after the fifth decade of life. If you're over age fifty and have a history of tobacco abuse, talk to your doctor about the possibility that emphysema is causing your symptoms.

How Your Doctor Can Help Find Your Asthma Triggers

I hope that by answering these questions, you now have a better idea about what triggers your asthma. I strongly suggest you speak to your doctor, who can be especially helpful in analyzing your asthma journal and testing you for other conditions (like GERD) that may be causing your symptoms. Ruling out medical conditions that can cause asthmalike symptoms is especially important, since some of you may be found not to have asthma at all. This is why it's so important to consider an alternative diagnosis and to get a second opinion. Even the best doctors get fooled and nobody can be right all the time. It never hurts to add a healthy dose of skepticism to any medical diagnosis.

Your doctor can also help you determine how much of your asthma is related to allergies. I suggest you ask your doctor about being tested for food, seasonal, and pet and dust-mite allergies. One caveat: Testing positive for a specific allergen does not mean this particular allergen is causing your asthma. Most asthmatics have multiple triggers and are sensitive to many different allergens. Testing positive does mean you are sensitive to a specific allergen that you should avoid in the future. In fact, avoiding allergens and asthma triggers whenever possible is without question the best way to treat asthma and will be the focus of Chapter 6: Home Decorating for the Asthmatic. Allergy testing is simply one more step on the way to making you asthma-free.

chapter 4

Healthy Living Boot Camp I: You Are What You Eat

I AM GOING TO ASK YOU TO DO the hardest thing in the world: to change how you live from day to day and to embrace healthy living. All I can do is advise—you have to decide how much you want to live and whether you're willing to change. If you want to live a full, rich life not tainted by illness or disability, read on. The following advice may save your life.

Another thing I must warn you about: Healthy living is hard. It requires commitment, which is especially difficult in a world filled with unhealthy temptations. Healthy living does not end six weeks from now, after your breathing returns to normal or you lose ten pounds. Healthy living is a way of life, seven days a week, twenty-four hours a day, for the rest of your life.

I hope you will be convinced that you can control your life and your asthma. However, I want you to be patient. Please don't try to change your life overnight. Too often people leave my office determined to do the right thing, desperate to make the changes as fast as they can. If you try to change too quickly, you'll only end up miserable the next day, missing all those things you once enjoyed. If you go from ice cream to celery sticks overnight, it will feel as if you've been sentenced to culinary purgatory. This is why diets and New Year's resolutions often fail. Permanent change occurs gradually, allowing you time to adjust. Remember, it took you a long time to get where you are and it will take time for you to change.

As you read this book, dedicate yourself to making and sticking with one healthy change every week. For instance, next week start eating fish every Monday night. The next week, in addition to Monday-night fish, start exercising every Wednesday morning. Then the next week, in addition to Monday fish and Wednesday exercise, start eating a high-fiber cereal with fresh fruit for breakfast every Saturday. This way, you make the changes gradually so they become a part of your everyday life. Over a period of three months, you won't believe how great you feel and how far you have come.

WHY TAKE CARE OF YOURSELF? THE REORGANIZATION OF MODERN HEALTHCARE

Let me tell you why I'm placing all the responsibility for your health and welfare on you. Not long ago, many people believed that modern medicine could cure almost anything. If you had a pain, you saw your doctor, who poked and prodded your tummy before handing you some pills and sending you off. You left nodding your head in appreciation. The reasons why this all-knowing doctor is becoming a thing of the past are complex. Over the last century, science and technology have made amazing strides, with new medical discoveries announced almost daily. From these unprecedented achievements grew a perception that any illness could be cured or, at the very least, controlled by a pill, a machine, or a surgeon's scalpel. Many people mistakenly believed that a pill could solve their problems like in television medical shows where everyone gets better in sixty minutes. At first, it seemed as if this was not too far from the truth. New, more powerful drugs were developed that were able to control, and even at times cure, some of our most devastating illnesses. People were still getting sick; however, now we could do something about it. It seemed like only a matter of time before science would eradicate all disease.

Then something interesting happened. People started living longer, a result of medical innovations and improved sanitation. The only problem was that with longer lives came a whole new set of medical problems—chronic, painful conditions like arthritis and fibromyalgia and deadly diseases like cancer, which despite some early encouraging victories are still winning the war. These illnesses were not only a consequence of advanced age, but problems that in many respects resulted from how and where people lived.

Modern medicine was ill prepared to deal with these new problems, because physicians (and patients) relied on technology to cure and treat illness. Few of our parents or grandparents were given advice on how to eat, sleep, or exercise. Rather, physicians waited for the disease to appear and then treated it with medicine or surgery. We are the product of generations of people who grew up believing that their health would be protected and preserved through modern medicine. People who were trained to rely on doctors for their health now comprise an elderly generation that has been tragically confronted by problems that cannot be cured with a simple pill or machine, problems that were caused in large part by unhealthy lifestyles.

Millions of Americans, after decades of fast food and sedentary lifestyles, are reaching their fifties and sixties crippled by ill health. Sure, doctors were able to prevent and treat many diseases, but nobody foresaw the consequences of keeping inactive people alive in a fast-food society. Nobody in the conventional medical community realized that if you don't keep the body fit, disaster is certain to follow with advancing age. As many of my patients have stated, "Yeah, I'm still alive, but I'm too old, sick, and tired to enjoy it!"

To further compound this tragedy, as the population aged, these conditions became more common. People flocked to their doctors, who could no longer give them the magic pill they so desperately desired. Not only did this essentially bankrupt the healthcare system, the psychological cost was devastating for people who had to face the fact that they were now stuck with their illness. They began to realize, "I'm not going to die from tuberculosis like my grandfather, but I'm going to spend the next thirty years weak, tired, and in pain." They felt betrayed by the healthcare system and especially by their doctors, dissatisfaction that was in part responsible for the upheavals we have witnessed in healthcare.

Yet, we can't blame doctors for failing to recognize that the most important thing a person can do is lay the foundation for lifelong health. We have to remember that the idea of healthy living has had a tumultuous history. For centuries, there were those who spoke about the benefits of leading a healthy and physically active life; however, when your average life expectancy is often no longer than thirty years, healthy living seems like a lot of work for little gain. It was not until the last hundred years or so, when life expectancy dramatically increased, that scientists began to take healthy living seriously. Even more telling, it has only been in the last forty years that researchers have aggressively investigated the impact of exercise, sleep, and diet on health and longevity. Modern medicine is finally changing and, like a phoenix rising from the ashes, a new, more mature approach to healthcare is emerging.

SCIENTIFIC RESEARCH AND SCIENTIFIC UNCERTAINTY

Some say that every particle of matter has an opposite, a piece of antimatter. The same can be said for many scientific studies; for every study that says X is true, there is another study that says Y is true and X is either wrong or was not as important as everyone thought. Controversy in science is good and keeps the research interesting, presenting new challenges that force our knowledge to grow. The public, however, as a rule is uneasy with the concept that uncertainty is a fact of scientific life.

Another important lesson is that no study is perfect. A decent statistician can find a flaw in almost any study. Many times researchers must make difficult decisions that can strengthen one part of a study at the expense of another. One problem we commonly see in research on nutritional supplements is that many early studies attempted to investigate the short-term effects of supplementation, an approach that often yields discouraging results. We now understand, however, that diet and supplements achieve their greatest benefit over months or years, not just a few days. Healthy living is a lifelong endeavor, not something to practice for a couple of weeks and discard once we feel or look better. As for asthma, we now know that healthy living works its magic not by aborting acute attacks but by preventing future attacks, something difficult to demonstrate in a research study.

There is also the whole subject of the relative strengths and weaknesses of different study designs, a subject that could easily fill several books. For our purposes, all research studies quoted in this book are subject to the same exacting standards and criticisms as any other type of scientific endeavor and display the same strengths and weaknesses inherent to all methods of inquiry.

Now, don't get me wrong, physicians do know a lot about the human body. Physicians know a lot about asthma and how to treat it, and few doctors would deny that allergies and asthma often go hand-in-hand. However, controversy rages on over how much allergies contribute to asthma. So, while there are many facts about asthma that most physicians agree on, there are many more unresolved questions that are subject to intense debate.

We also have to understand that scientists and physicians are trained to remain skeptical, to never accept anything at face value. For instance, it's not good enough that one study reports that vitamin C helps asthmatics. The "scientific method" demands that additional studies be performed to see if similar results can be achieved, a quality known as reproducibility. Reproducibility is central to the scientific method and is a major reason why controversy exists in medicine. It is also the reason why it often takes years for a particular finding to be accepted by the scientific community. Reproducibility is so important that, as far as the scientific method is concerned, there can be no facts without it.

Scientific discovery is not like a movie, with the wild-haired scientist surrounded by test tubes suddenly shouting, "Eureka!" Finding the truth is hard work and normally involves years of research coupled with persistent controversy. How we get to know what we know can be divided into three general stages: hypothesis, research-publication-controversy, and acceptance-rejection. This process of discovery can last decades, but it is the only way we can be remotely certain about the accuracy of scientific research.

What usually happens first is that someone reports an expected or unexpected finding in a study. From this new finding, a hypothesis is generated. For instance, a group of researchers are studying the relationship between diet and health and find that people with diets rich in fresh fruits have a lower risk of asthma. Another scientist reads their report and says to herself, "That's interesting. I know that fruits are rich in vitamin C and that vitamin C is a powerful antioxidant. I also know that oxidative stress plays a role in asthma. I wonder if giving asthmatics extra vitamin C will reduce their symptoms?" This is the hypothesis: Can vitamin C supplementation reduce asthma symptoms?

The researcher then designs a study to test her hypothesis. She develops a randomly controlled, double-blind study by giving half a group of asthmatics vitamin C and the other half a placebo. She then follows these two groups for a period of time, during which she measures several asthma-related variables like lung function and asthma severity scores. Once the study has been completed, the test results are compared between the two groups and presented to the scientific community, usually by being published in a scientific journal.

Other scientists see her report and decide to reproduce those results to determine if they're valid. This is where things get complicated. How a study is designed depends on the researcher and the type of data being collected. There are several basic study designs, each with their own strengths and weaknesses, and no two studies are exactly alike. As a result of these efforts, multiple studies examining the relationship between asthma and vitamin C begin to appear in the scientific literature. What often happens in early research is that some studies say vitamin C helps, some say vitamin C doesn't help, while other studies are inconclusive.

Researchers then critically review the published studies for flaws and design improved studies that they hope will yield reproducible results, a process that can take years to decades. This cycle of publication followed by critical review and additional publications is called the research-publication-controversy stage.

Ideally, over a period of years, what you find is a gradually evolving body of literature with more consistent findings. Once this occurs, we are at the acceptance-rejection part of the process. Yet, no matter how consistent the findings are among a group of papers, it is not uncommon to see newly published work that contradicts the established consensus. Sometimes these contradictory studies simply result from design flaws and are quickly dismissed. Other times, such studies represent the first step in toppling a medical dogma.

Throughout this book, as we examine integrative therapy research, we will see that some asthma therapies have more support than others. With some therapies, we may only be at the initial research stage with one or two published articles. With other therapies, there may be ten papers embroiled in controversy indicating the need for further studies. There will also be therapies that we'll be able to say with reasonable certainty that they work or don't work. I'll keep you apprised of where we are in the learning curve and how close we are to reaching a conclusion.

WHAT IS INTEGRATIVE MEDICINE?

Integrative medicine can perhaps best be defined as a way of preventing and treating disease using traditional and nontraditional therapies. Also known as alternative or complementary medicine, an increasing number of Americans are now embracing these practices and "integrating" them with conventional Western therapies. Multiple studies have documented that so-called alternative or complementary therapies are employed by a significant percentage of asthmatics. For instance, one survey found that 59 percent of 4,741 individuals with asthma had tried some form of integrative therapy, most commonly breathing therapy, homeopathy, and herbs.[1] In the United States, it is estimated that approximately 33 percent of the population has tried some form of complementary therapy; in Australia, this number approaches 50 percent.[2]

It will probably not surprise you to learn that integrative medicine continues to be shunned by many in the mainstream medical community. The good news is that integrative medicine is increasingly recognized by mainstream physicians as an important aspect of American medicine. Important not because millions of Americans practice some form of integrative medicine, but because some of these therapies work.

While many of these therapies, like traditional Chinese medicine, have been around for thousands of years, rigorous scientific research into integrative practices is only starting to emerge from its infancy. About forty years ago, scientists began to pay serious attention to diet and its impact on health, investigating this relationship both retrospectively and prospectively. In retrospective investigation, you search data you already have for a particular relationship. The best studies, however, are usually prospective, in which you collect new data and then examine it for a relationship.

Over the past twenty years, we have witnessed an explosion of publications that link diet to health. The overwhelming majority of physicians now believe that diet is intimately related to health. This does not mean that every disease can be blamed on diet, but rather that the scientific community recognizes that diet plays a pivotal role in many diseases. With respect to asthma, there are multiple published studies that have followed thousands of individuals for decades and demonstrate a definitive link between diet and asthma.

Once we have established that diet can influence asthma, the next logical question is, "What nutrient is responsible for this relationship? Is it vitamin C, zinc, selenium, or some yet unknown substance?" This is a critical question, for if we can find the specific nutrients that are active against asthma, we can use this knowledge to help people with asthma. We are now seeing multiple papers in the scientific literature that address this very issue.

The relationship between asthma and dietary supplements remains a topic of debate. Nevertheless, there are hundreds of excellent studies on integrative medicine produced by some of the most respected research institutions in the world. For some integrative therapies, there is excellent evidence supporting their use. For others, research is yielding mixed results, indicating the need for further studies. And for yet other integrative therapies, research has clearly failed to support their effectiveness.

A NEW ERA: THE DOCTOR-PATIENT CONTRACT

Our emerging knowledge of diet and asthma opens new avenues for asthma management. Perhaps the most profound impact of dietary research is that it forces us to think about who is ultimately responsible for our health: is it the doctor, the patient, or both? Physicians and patients are starting to realize that healthcare is a two-way street. Up until recently, most healthcare professionals placed too much emphasis on treating asthma after the disease had already caused problems. Mercifully, this attitude is rapidly changing. We are beginning to realize that most diseases are preventable and their expression represents a failure of the healthcare system.

All too often, I see men and women who by their thirties have already racked up an impressive list of medical problems, like diabetes and hypertension. The bitter truth is that most of these individuals do not take care of themselves. They have horrendous diets, they religiously avoid exercise but will not miss a day of smoking or drinking, and they are all almost invariably overweight. This sad scenario represents a failure of the patients, for not taking care of themselves, and a failure of the healthcare system, for not hammering home the message that most illnesses are preventable. If it weren't for smoking, alcohol, fast food, lack of exercise, and unsafe sex, most doctors would be out of work. There simply would not be enough heart disease, asthma, diabetes, or hypertension to keep them employed.

As a society, we are beginning to realize that prevention is the essence of health and the responsibility of both doctors and patients. The cornerstone of prevention is adopting and maintaining a healthy lifestyle. This does not mean that healthy living will prevent every illness. Remember, disease results from a complex interplay between genes and environment and some people just have bad genes. This is why you occasionally read about someone who regularly runs marathons and suddenly dies from a heart attack. However, this is an exceedingly rare occurrence and only makes the news because it is so uncommon and unexpected. One truth remains: For the overwhelming majority of people, healthy living translates into a healthy, long, and active life.

How can healthy living aid the asthmatic? In addition to helping you avoid illness, healthy living can make your asthma either disappear or become much more manageable. In fact, adopting a healthy lifestyle can help most any medical problem. Diabetes and hypertension can disappear or improve dramatically through simple weight loss and diet. The same is true of asthma. Many people who embrace healthy living will either rid themselves of asthma or, at the very least, make their asthma infinitely more tolerable. Ridding yourself of asthma rests on three pillars: exercise, lifestyle modification, and a healthy, asthma-friendly diet. With that said, let's jump right into diet and see what you have to eat to beat asthma.

DIET: EAT TO LIVE LONGER, NOT TO LOSE WEIGHT

"Diet" is a four-letter word. Just looking at the word "diet" is distasteful, as I conjure up images of eating granola and tree bark. But "diet" doesn't always have to be a four-letter word; a healthy diet can be tasty and satisfying. Fundamentally, what I'm asking you to do is, over a period of months, gradually shift your diet from a meat-loving, fatty Western diet to a healthier, fish and vegetable-rich diet. You don't have to give up everything—you can still have the occasional steak and pint of ice cream—just eat less of them.

I'm not going to tell you what percentage of your diet should come from fat, protein, and carbohydrates. Nor will I suggest how many calories you should eat every day. Rather than focusing your attention on minutia, concentrate on healthy living, on *what* you're eating, not how much. Concern yourself on how you exercise and how you feel, not on how many minutes you pound the treadmill or how many calories you burn off. Counting calories only forces you to fixate on food. Rather, your focus should be devoted to lifestyle, asking yourself every day "What have I done today to make my life better?" not "How many calories does this slice of cheese have?" If, after three months, you still haven't achieved a slimmer and healthier you, then I might recommend visiting a nutritionist to talk about calories and carbohydrates.

Diet is extremely important for anyone with a medical condition, especially asthma. Multiple studies have documented that a healthy diet can protect against asthma, whereas an unhealthy diet can increase the risk of asthma. For many asthmatics, eating right will mean the difference between feeling lousy and feeling well. For some asthmatics, diet may mean the difference between life and death, a message demonstrated by a British study that linked high salt intake to increased asthma mortality.[3]

Too many people confuse diet with weight loss. The advice given in this chapter has nothing to do with weight loss, and I rarely talk about weight loss with my patients. Rather, I emphasize that if you eat a healthy diet and exercise, weight loss will happen by itself. The problem with focusing on weight loss is that it fixates you on a goal, such as losing ten pounds. Know what happens to people who think like this? Once they've met their goal, they forget about the diet and pack those pounds right back on. Weight loss forces people to think in the short-term. Healthy living, on the other hand, helps you think about the rest of your life.

WHY EAT A HEALTHY DIET? THE IMPORTANCE OF ANTIOXIDANTS

A healthy diet is vital for everyone, not just asthmatics, and eating right can protect you from high blood pressure, cancer, high cholesterol, allergies, and a host of other ills. Diet does this primarily by supplying the body with vital nutrients that permit normal function and boost the immune system. More important for asthmatics, a healthy diet provides an ample supply of antioxidants, critical weapons against the oxidative stress that is in part responsible for initiating the asthma cascade.

Some studies even point to dietary factors such as inadequate antioxidant intake for the increasing incidence of asthma. In one British study examining the effects of diet on asthma, the researchers state that "the observed reduction in antioxidant intake in the British diet over the last twenty-five years has been a factor in the increase in the prevalence of asthma over this period." The authors write that "populations of economically advanced countries have eaten a diet which has included less fresh fruit and vegetables and this diet has increased the susceptibility to potentially harmful, inhaled substances by reducing the antioxidant defenses of the lung against the effects of inhaled irritants and allergens." They conclude that diet has an important protective role to play in the prevention of bronchial reactivity.[4] This sentiment is echoed by multiple studies that have concluded that people with asthma often have diets poor in antioxidants.

What exactly do we mean when we use the word "oxidation"? In nature, two basic types of chemical reactions occur: oxidation and reduction. Oxidation happens when a molecule loses electrons, whereas reduction occurs when a molecule gains electrons. When a molecule is oxidized, it becomes a free radical, a highly reactive and unstable molecule that can damage and kill the cells in your body. Free radicals are blamed for many of our most devastating diseases, including heart disease, diabetes, and asthma. If free radicals left us alone, we'd probably live a lot longer and wouldn't get very sick.

Because nature prefers stability, this unstable free radical attempts to regain its former stability by stealing electrons from another molecule, which itself then becomes an unstable and reactive free radical. This losing and gaining of electrons results in a chain reaction of multiple free radicals generating more free radicals. These oxidation-reduction chain reactions occur in our bodies every day and are usually well controlled by our own antioxidants, biochemical molecules that neutralize free radicals. In fact, a small amount of oxidative reactions are needed to protect our health, as free radicals are routinely employed by our immune system to kill microorganisms. Problems occur when our antioxidant forces are overwhelmed, allowing free radicals to wreak havoc on our tissues and organs, a condition known as oxidative stress.

While everyone would be better off if they could avoid oxidative stress, free radicals are a fact of life. The body's chief defenses against oxidative stress are antioxidants, which come in two primary forms: water soluble and fat soluble. Glutathione and vitamin C are two key water-soluble antioxidants; vitamin E and the carotenoids belong to the fat-soluble group.

Perhaps one of the easiest ways to understand oxidants and antioxidants is from the perspective of supply and demand. On the supply side, as we age our antioxidant reserves dwindle, permitting the ravages of aging and disease to take hold. Poor nutrition can also devastate our antioxidant defenses, since the body is heavily dependent on dietary sources of antioxidants. An unhealthy diet can deplete our antioxidant reserves, leading to oxidative damage and subsequent disease. On the demand side, anything that puts stress on the body can increase free radicals. This stress can be caused by a medical condition or environmental pollutants. In fact, environmental oxidative stress is now believed to be a leading contributor to the rising incidence of many diseases, including cancer.

Oxidative stress and antioxidants play a dramatic role in asthma. Asthma is a state of chronic airway inflammation, with inflammatory cells releasing free radicals that exacerbate the vicious cycle of asthma. Specifically, free radicals are blamed for bronchospasm, excess mucus production, and histamine release, all essential features of asthma. Not only do free radicals play a leading role in asthma, it appears that the free radicals produced by asthmatics are more toxic than those in people without asthma.

Without question, asthma is associated with an imbalance of free radicals that leads to increased oxidant stress.[5] This is why the major emphasis of conventional medical therapy is directed at reducing inflammation and why, for better or worse, steroids are effective in treating asthma. From a natural-remedy perspective, this is why there is increasing interest in the role antioxidants play in the prevention and treatment of asthma. It is hoped that antioxidant nutrients and supplements can reduce inflammation without the potentially harmful side effects found with drugs.

In addition to protecting the body from internal oxidative stress, antioxidants play a major role in protecting the lungs from external harm. The United States has major air pollution problems, which many authorities believe are partly responsible for the current asthma epidemic. There are thousands of toxins released into the atmosphere daily, many of which can increase the lung's oxidative load, with the potential to exacerbate asthma. Building our antioxidant reserves can help prevent lung damage by attenuating this toxic insult.

For an asthmatic, the logic for boosting antioxidants goes like this: More antioxidants translate into fewer free radicals, which translates into reduced lung damage and irritation and fewer asthmatic symptoms. Supporting the role antioxidants play in fighting asthma are multiple studies that demonstrate impaired lung function in individuals who eat fewer fruits and vegetables, foods rich in natural antioxidants. One study of 2,650 European children, from the St. George's Hospital Medical School in London, examined the effect of fresh fruit consumption on FEV_1 (Forced Expiratory Volume in One Second) and found that "FEV_1 was positively associated with frequency of fresh fruit consumption." The study also reported that children who never ate fresh fruit had an estimated FEV_1 that was 4.3 percent lower than those who ate fruit more than once daily. The authors concluded that fresh fruit appeared to be beneficial for lung function in children.[6]

Other studies have linked low fruit consumption to poor lung function. One study from England examined the effect of fruit and fruit juice consumption on lung function in nearly 3,000 adults, ages eighteen to sixty-nine. The researchers found that the mean FEV_1 among those who never drank fresh fruit juice and ate fresh fruit less than once a week was significantly lower than among those who had higher levels of fruit consumption. The authors concluded that "these results support the hypothesis of an association between infrequent fruit or fruit juice consumption and impaired ventilatory function in adults."[7]

Another group of researchers from the University of Auckland in New Zealand, examined data from fifty-three nations that participated in the International Study of Asthma and Allergies in Childhood (ISAAC). The researchers found that there was "a consistent pattern of decreases in the symptoms of wheeze (current and severe), allergic rhinoconjunctivitis, and atopic eczema, associated with increased consumption of calories from cereal and rice, protein from cereal and nuts, starch, as well as vegetables and vegetable nutrients." The authors concluded that if the average daily consumption of these foods increased, an important decrease in symptoms could be achieved.[8] In other words, eat a healthy diet and your asthma symptoms will probably get better—simple as that!

Having established that diet, and especially antioxidants, play a major role in alleviating asthma and maintaining overall health, let's examine the impact foods have on how we breathe.

FRUITS AND VEGETABLES 101

Good old-fashioned fruits and vegetables can help solve some very modern problems. Besides tasting as good as they look, we are now learning that many of your standard vegetable-patch residents can help fight the war against cancer, heart disease, high cholesterol, and yes—even asthma. The best thing about these colorful characters is that you don't have to go to a health food store or doctor to get them.

Carotenoids (or Carotenes)

Remember when you were a child and your mother told you to eat your vegetables? Mom was onto something: Vegetables and fruits, especially those brightly colored ones, are rich in substances called carotenoids. Carotenoids are important not only because they give your salads and fruits those wonderful colors, but also because they fight cancer and are potent antioxidants that can protect you against asthma. In fact, the reason why plants make carotenoids is to protect themselves from free radicals. So, whenever you hear the word "vegetable" or "fruit," a smile should come to your face and the word "good" should fall from your lips.

There are about 600 different carotenoids, but only fourteen of these fat-soluble compounds concern the well-being of humans, with most of the excitement over five in particular—alpha-carotene, beta-carotene, lycopene, lutein, and zeaxanthin. Besides being important for lung health, these carotenoids play important roles in preventing heart disease, cataracts, and macular degeneration. Asthmatics tend to get shortchanged when it comes to antioxidants, and studies have found that many asthmatics are deficient in beta-carotene. Even worse, decreased dietary beta-carotene may increase cancer risk and cardiovascular disease. Besides protecting our lungs from oxidative stress, carotenoids are essential for making vitamin A, which is needed for a healthy immune system. This is especially important for asthmatics considering that viral infections can cause asthma exacerbations.

That carotenoids play an important role in immune function is an accepted fact, but whether or not carotenoids enhance immune function independently or through vitamin A remains controversial. There is, however, evidence that dietary beta-carotene independently boosts immune function and protects against cancer. It's probably better to let the scientists sort this out while you just eat your vegetables. The important message is that carotenoids can help your asthma, in particular by protecting you against viral infections, which can make an asthmatic's life miserable.

One Israeli randomized, double-blind, placebo-controlled trial of thirty-eight patients with exercise-induced asthma (EIA) examined the effect of giving the subjects 64 mg of natural beta-carotene per day. The study found that 53 percent of the subjects who took beta-carotene "were protected against EIA."[9] Another study from the same group examined the effect of supplementing with lycopene (30 mg daily) in twenty patients with EIA for one week. In the lycopene group, 55 percent of the patients were significantly protected against EIA, most probably through an antioxidative effect, according to the authors.[10]

Alpha-Carotene

Alpha-carotene is abundant in carrots and leafy green vegetables. Most authorities recommend at least 6.5 mg of alpha-carotene a day. Drug interactions with bile-acid sequestrants and colestipol are reported, so talk to your doctor before supplementing with alpha-carotene if you're taking any of these medications.

Beta-Carotene

Beta-carotene is found in broccoli, cantaloupe, carrots, pink grapefruit, sweet potatoes, and virtually all leafy green vegetables. While there are no official guidelines for carotenoid intake, the typical daily dose of 15 mg (or 25,000 IU) of natural beta-carotene a day is a good start.

I emphasize "natural" beta-carotene because studies have suggested that smokers (especially smokers who drink alcohol) who take synthetic beta-carotene may actually increase their risk of lung cancer. If you smoke, avoid synthetic beta-carotene supplements and stick with good old-fashioned fruits and vegetables. Another reason to avoid synthetic beta-carotene is that it does not pack the antioxidant punch found in the natural product.

If you decide to take additional beta-carotene, stick to naturally derived sources that come from *Dunaliella salina* algae. Don't go overboard with beta-carotene, since doses over 30 mg a day can turn your skin yellow-orange; this side effect is reversible by stopping supplementation. You should also take additional vitamin E, as prolonged beta-carotene supplementation may reduce vitamin E levels. As for drug interactions, beta-carotene can react with bile-acid sequestrants, cisplatin, colchicine, colestipol, cyclophosphamide, docetaxel, lansoprazole, methyltestosterone, mineral oil, neomycin, orlistat, paclitaxel, quinidine, and chemotherapy drugs. Check with your doctor before supplementing with beta-carotene if you're taking any of these medications.

Lycopene

To boost lycopene levels, eat plenty of apricots, carrots, green peppers, and tomatoes. Tomato paste and sauce are particularly rich sources of lycopene, a carotenoid antioxidant that appears to be more powerful than beta-carotene and is known to protect against a variety of diseases, including prostate cancer. There is also evidence that lycopene can protect against heart disease and boost immune function. Most authorities recommend at least 6.5 mg of lycopene per day. No drug interactions have been reported with lycopene.

Lutein

Lutein-rich foods include corn, carrots, potatoes, spinach, lettuce, peas, egg yolks, tomatoes, and any leafy green vegetable. Typically, take at least 6 mg of lutein daily. No drug interactions have been reported with lutein.

Zeaxanthin

Leafy green vegetables are particularly rich in zeaxanthin. Most authorities recommend 6 mg of zeaxanthin daily.

When shopping for fruits and vegetables, as a general rule remember that the more intense the color, the greater the concentration of carotenoids. A final word about cooking: Although carotenoids do not degrade with cooking, given the fact that cooking may destroy other vital nutrients, I recommend steaming your vegetables or eating them raw. Most authorities recommend, at a minimum, five to six fruit and vegetable servings daily.

Flavonoids

Flavonoids (or bioflavonoids) are water-soluble pigments found in plants that are important antioxidants and aid in the absorption of vitamin C. Originally called vitamin P, these substances include citrin, epicatechin, flavones, flavonols, hesperidin, quercetin, and rutin. While there is some debate over how to classify flavonoids, most authorities agree that they possess a variety of antihistamine, anti-inflammatory, antioxidant, and anti-viral activities. Because of these characteristics, flavonoids are used to treat blood vessel disorders, diabetes, night blindness, and minor injuries.

Popular flavonoids include quercetin, found in onions, and genistein, commonly found in soy. Flavonoids are also found in wine, tea, apples, and citrus fruits. Apparently, an apple a day does keep the doctor away, according to a study from King's College, London, on the dietary habits of 9,709 individuals. The results, published in the *American Journal of Respiratory and Critical Care Medicine* in 2001, showed that people who ate two or more apples a week reduced their asthma risk by 28 percent.[11]

Quercetin is structurally similar to the allergy drug disodium cromoglycate and boasts a variety of anti-inflammatory and antioxidant effects, which is why it is useful for treating asthma. Perhaps even more important, there is evidence that quercetin inhibits leukotrienes and blocks histamine release. As you may recall, leukotrienes are a major contributor to the asthma cascade and some of the most effective asthma drugs work by inhibiting leukotrienes. There are presently no human studies on quercetin and asthma, but animal studies support the antiasthmatic action of this flavonoid.

Mixed Flavonoids

As with the carotenoids, the best offense is a good defense—so, do as your mother said and eat your fruits and vegetables. Several flavonoid supplements are also available, and most authorities recommend 1,000 mg of citrus flavonoids daily. As for drug interactions, flavonoids can react with acyclovir, so check with your doctor before supplementing if you're taking this medicine.

Quercetin

Found in apples, beans, green and black tea, onions, and many leafy green vegetables, quercetin is used in the treatment of capillary disorders, arteriosclerosis, asthma, and diabetes. For asthmatics, the standard dose of quercetin is 400 mg two to three times a day. Side effects have not been reported; however, since quercetin can cause chromosomal abnormalities in bacteria, women who plan to become or are pregnant should not take quercetin. If you decide to supplement your diet, use quercetin chalcone, a water-soluble form that is more easily absorbed. Since quercetin can react with estradiol and felodipine, check with your doctor before supplementing if you are taking these medicines.

More Reasons to Eat Your Fruits and Vegetables

Fruits and vegetables contain not only asthma-friendly carotenoids and flavonoids, but are also packed with vital nutrients, such as vitamins A, C, and E, which play a critical role in preventing and treating asthma. With fruits and veggies, variety is the spice of life. I'm not going to bias you by recommending a particular veggie or fruit, as they all have their merits. What I suggest is that, every other day, you try a different vegetable or fruit and settle on those that appeal to your taste buds. One night, you can eat a dish of asparagus, while the next night you might have some yellow peppers with onions. Try not to exile your vegetables to a side dish, but rather include them in your nightly salad and entrée. For instance, try halibut topped with a mixture of finely chopped red and yellow peppers with onions. The tension between the rather bland halibut and the zesty peppers and onions will leave you begging for more. The possibilities are endless and entire cookbooks are devoted to fruits and vegetables.

Remember, vegetables are best served steamed or raw, because these methods preserve the nutrients and enhance the flavor. Bottom line: Vegetables do not have to be boring or taste bad, so eat your vegetables!

MEAT OR FISH?

Many people see meat and fish as dietary archenemies, competing against each other like matter and antimatter or good versus evil. What if I said that you can have your meat and eat it too? There's nothing wrong with a little meat; I just want you to eat more fish and less meat. One of the primary factors in recommending a diet with smaller amounts of meat is fat. There are good fats and bad fats, and meat tends to contain the bad fats, whereas fish usually contains the good fats. One study from Taiwan found a link between asthma and consuming meat, with teenagers who ate meat or liver having over 1.5 times the risk of asthma.[12]

Fish are frequently rich in omega-3 fatty acids, a type of fat that may improve your lung function and help you live longer. Just to give you a taste of the benefits of eating fish, one Harvard study examined the dietary habits of 84,688 women and found that those who ate fish two to four times a week decreased their risk of heart disease by 31 percent.[13] Several studies also demonstrate that the more fish you consume, the better your lung function and the lower your risk of asthma, a finding that appears to be strongest in children. One Australian study examined the effect of consuming oily fish—defined as fish containing greater than 2 percent fat—in 574 children. Researchers found that children who ate oily fish more than once a week had a 75 percent reduction in asthma risk.[14]

Another Harvard study examined the diets of 2,526 adults who took part in the First National Health and Nutritional Examination Survey (NHANES I). These scientists reported that high fish consumption had a "protective association with FEV_1." Specifically, they found a 115 milliliter difference in FEV_1 between those eating fish less than once a week and those eating fish more than once a week.[15] The authors concluded that dietary intake of fish is associated with higher levels of lung function.[16]

Another study from Italy found that 3 grams of fish oil a day for thirty days reduced bronchial hyperreactivity and residual volume (RV) in people with seasonal allergic asthma. RV is the amount of air left in the lung after you exhale, which can increase dramatically during an asthma attack. Specifically, the authors measured FEV_1 and Raw, a measure of airway resistance, before and after fish-oil supplementation. Prior to treatment, the maximal drop in FEV_1 was 28 percent, whereas after supplementation the maximal drop was 11 percent. Similar results were reported for Raw, which was 265 percent prior to supplementation, plummeting to 37 percent after treatment.[17]

These studies offer encouraging evidence regarding the impact a healthy diet has on asthma. As in all scientific endeavors, especially those that examine the effects of diet on a medical condition, there are conflicting studies; however, this should not dissuade asthmatics from increasing their fish consumption. Considering the important role fish oils play in preserving overall health, eating fish is a win-win situation.

Of course, there are exceptions. Some farm-raised fish are bred to have a higher "bad" fat content to improve taste (and sales), but they are simply fatty fish. Included on the list of farm-raised fatty fish are salmon, trout, and catfish. So, before you plunk down a hunk of money for "healthy" fish, ask your grocer where the fish hails from. Wild fish, with their higher concentrations of omega-3 fatty acids, give you the most bang (more healthy fat) for your fish buck.

Like fish, not all meats are of equal nutritional value. There is little question that meat contains vital proteins and nutrients. What you want to do with all your food choices is gain as much nutritional value as possible with a minimum amount of fat. In this regard, chicken and game meats are better choices. Chicken, especially without the skin, has much less fat than the average steak. If you can't live without red meat, consider naturally lean meats like venison and ostrich, which pack a low-fat but high-nutritional punch. Adding steak or barbecue sauce will do wonders to improve the flavor of these low-fat game meats. If you can't find game at your local grocery store, ask your grocer about availability. There are also several websites that, for a few spare bucks (pun intended), will ship you all the game you want. If you insist on beef, buy lean cuts and have the excess fat trimmed away.

NOT ALL FATS ARE CREATED EQUAL

Who doesn't like fat? Fat makes food taste great and perhaps millions of years ago eating lots of fat conferred a survival advantage. Pound for pound, fat packs the most energy per unit consumed. The only problem is that we no longer need that energy to hunt for food or run from hostile tribes, so all that fat goes to our thighs, bellies, and arteries.

Polyunsaturated fatty acids—omega-3s and omega-6s—are what we call "good" fats. You want to avoid saturated fats, which are commonly found in baked goods like donuts and potato chips. And completely avoid margarine and other hydrogenated oils. These contain trans-fatty acids, a synthetic type of saturated fat that is far worse for your heart than butter. Trans-fatty acids also interfere with the normal metabolism of heart-friendly omega-3 and omega-6 fatty acids.

Besides protecting your heart, avoiding fat is in your best interest. There is an emerging body of evidence that increased fat intake may be contributing to the asthma epidemic. One study from Sweden examined 478 men and found that "men with asthma had a significantly higher intake of fat than men without asthma."[18] Another study from Taiwan examined the diets of 1,166 teenagers and found that those with a high intake of saturated fats had twice the risk of asthma, whereas intake of monounsaturated fats decreased the risk by approximately 35 percent.[19]

As you've seen, there is increasing evidence that high fish intake can protect against asthma. Fish work their magic through essential fatty acids (fish oils)—"essential" because our bodies can't make them and we have to rely on dietary sources—such as alpha-linolenic acid (omega-3) and linoleic acid (omega-6). Fish oils are also heart friendly, helping to lower triglycerides and keeping atherosclerosis in check. Because of their anti-inflammatory properties, fish oils are used to treat a number of conditions, such as high blood pressure and diabetes. The chief omega-3 fatty acids are eicosapentaenoic acid (EPA) and docosahexaenoic acid (DHA), which can be found in a variety of fish including anchovies, albacore tuna, herring, sardines, and salmon. Omega-3s are also found in flaxseed oil, walnut oil, game meat, and that old favorite, cod liver oil.

While omega-6 is a healthy fat, too much omega-6 may actually increase your risk of heart disease and high blood pressure. Some experts even suspect that excess omega-6 may make asthma worse. Researchers hypothesize that our increased consumption of omega-6s, coupled with decreased intake of omega-3s, is partly responsible for the rising incidence of asthma. Omega-6 is under suspicion because it is used by the body to make arachidonic acid, which in turn can be converted to prostaglandin E_2 (PGE_2) and leukotrienes, two major players in the asthma cascade. Conversely, EPA and DHA are known to inhibit PGE_2 and leukotriene synthesis. Far from settled, this controversy should not cause you to avoid fish or omega-6s. I strongly recommend that you maintain a healthy balance between the omega-3s and omega-6s, since these fats are essential to your health.

SUPPLEMENTING WITH HEALTHY FATS

For supplementation, most authorities typically recommend 10 grams of fish oil, daily. Some experts go a little higher, suggesting 2–9 grams of omega-3s and 9–18 grams of omega-6s. You can meet these requirements simply by mixing a tablespoon of flaxseed oil with your favorite food, daily. Always remember to maintain a healthy balance between omega-3s and omega-6s in order to avoid increasing your risk of heart disease and possibly exacerbating your asthma.

Nutritional experts also recommend washing fish oil down with an antioxidant, like vitamin E, to preserve the potency of the oil, which is extremely sensitive to oxygen degradation. Side effects are uncommon but can include stomach upset, which can be avoided by taking "enteric-coated" supplements. Since fish oil can, on rare occasions, raise LDL cholesterol, anyone with heart disease or high cholesterol should talk to his or her doctor before taking supplements. The same is true for individuals with diabetes, since fish oil can potentially raise blood sugar. There is some evidence that this undesirable effect on blood sugar can be prevented by taking vitamin E or by exercising regularly (three times a week).

Consult a doctor if you are pregnant and plan on taking essential fatty acid supplements. Also, speak to your physician if you intend to regularly take cod liver oil that contains over 25,000 IU of vitamin A or over 800 IU of vitamin D. As for drug interactions, since fish and cod liver oil can react with cyclosporine, pravastatin, and simvastatin, check with your doctor before supplementing if you are taking these medications. Also, if you have aspirin-sensitive asthma, talk to your physician before taking fish oils, as they may reduce lung function in this type of asthmatic.

Healthy omega-3 and omega-6 cooking oils include canola, flaxseed, hemp, and walnut oil. When I cook, in addition to using my favorite heart-friendly oil, I use wine. Wine adds flavor and helps keep food from burning, thereby allowing you to use less butter and oil. Try to maintain a healthy balance between omega-3 and omega-6 fatty acids by using a different cooking oil each time you prepare a meal. Remember, omega-3s and omega-6s are the good fats and may protect you against asthma.

A VEGETARIAN DIET FOR ASTHMA?

There is something to be said for not eating meat on philosophical grounds; however, even more important for our purposes, a vegetarian diet is clearly a healthy diet. Much to my amazement, I could only find one scientific study examining the impact of a vegetarian diet on asthma. This study followed thirty-five medication-dependent asthmatics who consumed a vegan diet with no meat, fish, eggs, tea (herbal teas were allowed), chocolate, sugar, coffee, and milk for one year. According to the authors, there was a significant decrease in asthma symptoms and, in almost all cases, medication was stopped or drastically reduced. After four months, 71 percent of the participants reported reduced symptoms or no symptoms, with the percentage increasing to 92 percent after one year. The authors also reported decreases in weight, blood pressure, and heart rate. Plus, FEV_1 rose from an average of 2.0 L to 2.5 L, with an increase in vital capacity from 3.4 L to 4.0 L after one year.[20] Vital capacity, the amount of air you can fully exhale, is an especially important measure of lung function for asthmatics, since asthma is characterized by air trapping (not being able to get all the air out of the lungs).

While this study clearly demonstrates that a vegetarian diet can help people with asthma, more studies are needed. After reviewing the literature on diet and asthma and taking into consideration the vital role antioxidants play, I strongly recommend a vegetarian diet to anyone who can tolerate it. A vegetarian diet may or may not "cure" your asthma but, at the very least, it will help you to live a longer, healthier life. As with eating fish, you can't lose by being a vegetarian—it's a win-win situation.

The truth, however, about vegetarianism is that not everyone (myself included) can live without meat, fish, and dairy products. I strike a personal balance by rarely eating meat, with most of my evening meals consisting of fish. I try to eat vegetarian for breakfast and lunch whenever possible. Vegetarians should remember to supplement their diet with vitamin B_{12}, calcium, vitamin D, iron, selenium, and zinc, since the lack of meat, fish, or dairy products can translate into several vitamin and mineral deficiencies. Taking a daily multivitamin helps prevent these deficiencies.

CAFFEINE

Some people can't live with it, others can't live without it. A central nervous-system stimulant, caffeine can alleviate asthma symptoms. Caffeine contains methylxanthine, the same active ingredient found in the drug theophylline. Caffeine's impact on asthma is dose dependent, which means the more you drink, the better you feel.

One US Environmental Protection Agency study found that people who regularly drank coffee reduced their risk of asthma symptoms by 29 percent.[21] An Italian group examined data from 72,284 individuals and concluded that "caffeine intake had a bronchodilatory effect in asthma." The study indirectly suggested that long-term, moderate coffee consumption may reduce symptoms and also prevent bronchial asthma. Specifically, they found that a daily cup of coffee reduced asthma risk by 5 percent and that three cups daily reduced risk by 28 percent.[22] One randomized, placebo-controlled trial examined the effect of high-dose caffeine (7 mg/kg of body weight) on exercise-induced asthma. The authors found that caffeine significantly improved FEV_1 and prevented exercise-induced bronchoconstriction.[23]

One study found that caffeine (at a dose of 5 mg/kg of body weight) can produce significant improvement in objective measures of lung function in adult asthmatics. The authors reported an average 17 percent improvement in FEV_1 after caffeine ingestion.[24] Finally, the Cochrane database reports that "caffeine appears to improve airway function modestly in people with asthma for up to four hours."[25]

Caffeine's antiasthma effects begin approximately one hour after ingestion and last up to six hours. Most authorities recommend 350 mg of caffeine daily for asthmatics. Since the average eight-ounce cup of coffee contains 135–150 mg of caffeine, most people need two to three cups of coffee, daily, to achieve an adequate bronchodilatory response. You can also get your caffeine kick from tea; however, since tea contains about half the caffeine of coffee, you just have to drink more of it. Caffeine doesn't come without a price and can increase your risk of insomnia, anxiety, osteoporosis, and abnormal heart rhythms. People who take theophylline should exercise caution regarding caffeine intake, as both have side effects that are additive.

SALT

Salt (sodium) is everywhere in the food supply; you just can't escape it. If you love salt—and who doesn't?—the news is not good. Since 1938, high sodium intake has been associated with asthma. As with many studies on diet and asthma, the role salt plays in asthma remains controversial. Several authors do, however, blame increased salt intake for the fact that asthma is more common in affluent nations than in less-developed countries. In fact, one study suggested that asthma deaths in men were related to elevated salt intake. Studies have also demonstrated that high-salt diets can increase airway reactivity. One study from the Catholic University in Rome examined salt consumption among 2,593 subjects and concluded that "personal table salt use is related to an increased prevalence of bronchial symptoms."[26]

But these studies are not conclusive. In 2002, The Cochrane Library issued a report entitled "Dietary Salt Reduction or Exclusion for Allergic Asthma," which reviewed multiple studies on salt intake and asthma. The report stated that "based on currently available evidence, it is not possible to conclude whether dietary salt reduction has any place in the treatment or management of asthma."[27] In other words, we need more studies.

There is emerging evidence that a strong relationship exists between salt and exercise-induced asthma (EIA). One double-blind, crossover study of nine men and six women found that a low-salt diet improved lung function, whereas a high-salt intake exacerbated EIA.[28] This conclusion was confirmed by another group that found that salt and chloride worsened EIA symptoms after a normal or high-salt diet.[29]

Given the negative health effects of excess salt in addition to the real possibility that salt can exacerbate asthma, I strongly suggest that asthmatics abstain from excess salt. Maintain a low-salt diet not only to protect your lungs, but also to avoid high blood pressure, stroke, heart disease, stomach cancer, and osteoporosis—conditions linked to high-salt intake. Be smart and cut back on the salt.

A FINAL WORD ON DIET

I debated whether or not to discuss how to calculate the calories you need to stay alive or to lose weight. Personally, I don't believe in counting calories because it reminds me of that four-letter word "diet." If you really need to lose weight, the last thing you want to do is starve yourself. People who starve themselves and rapidly lose excess pounds are destined to regain even more weight. This is why diets fail miserably!

As far as our bodies are concerned, we are metabolically still living in the time of saber-toothed tigers, when it was literally feast or famine with the food supply. Starvation makes your body respond as if there is a famine; it doesn't know you're just dieting. So, believing your life is in jeopardy, your body tries to hang on to every calorie it can by storing those calories as fat. This is why rapid weight loss only sets people up for failure: when they stop the weight-loss program, they inevitably gain back the weight they lost.

Though I hate to use the phrase "lose weight," over 50 percent of Americans have a weight problem so we might as well talk about it. To really lose weight, you have to stop trying to lose weight. Concentrate your efforts on healthy living and the weight loss will happen by itself. You should never starve yourself, because starvation only tells your body to start packing on the fat. Eat three satisfying healthy meals a day and avoid snacking between meals. Depending on how much weight you need to lose, give yourself six months to two years to achieve an ideal weight. The most successful weight loss occurs slowly, allowing your body to adapt to a trimmer you. Also, talk to your doctor or another qualified healthcare professional about weight loss.

If you want to calculate your ideal weight, use the following formulas:

- Ideal Body Weight for Men: 110 pounds + 5 pounds per inch over five feet tall
- Ideal Body Weight for Women: 100 pounds + 5 pounds per inch over five feet tall

While this is an "ideal" target weight, a variation of five to ten pounds in either direction can still be considered normal weight.

Although I do not advocate counting calories, I do recommend you read food labels, which give you information on calories and percentages of recommended daily fat per serving. For instance, if a serving has 50 percent of the recommended fat, the food is clearly fattening. Conversely, a product with only 2 percent of the daily fat is probably less fattening. Once again, you have to be careful of some "fat-free" products that have absolutely no fat but, to improve taste, are loaded with salt or 300 calories of pure sugar. The lesson here is that you should be suspicious of foods that claim to be "low-fat" or "fat-free." Some manufacturers make this claim but load their products with fat-forming sugars or make their portions unreasonably small. Remember, when reading food labels, pay attention to calories and fat per portion, as well as portion size.

The honest calculus of weight loss is that you must burn more calories than you consume, a feat that is nearly impossible to do safely through diet alone. To successfully lose those pounds, you need to speed up your body's metabolic rate so your cells burn more calories. The best way to do this is through exercise. In fact, a healthy diet combined with regular exercise is the best and only way to achieve permanent weight loss. Even better news: Exercise may also help your asthma and allow you to live a longer and healthier life.

chapter 5

Healthy Living Boot Camp II: Exercise, Sleep, and Eliminating Bad Habits

NOW THAT WE'VE COVERED DIET, let's examine some of the other aspects of a healthy lifestyle that can play a critical role in alleviating asthma. First on the list is exercise, something asthmatics should learn to embrace, not fear. Not only is regular exercise good for overall health, but it can also improve your asthma. Getting enough sleep—something easier said than done in many cases—is also important. Sleep rejuvenates the immune system and is critical to general health. Finally, giving up smoking, excessive drinking, and illegal drugs is vital to living with asthma.

ASTHMA AND EXERCISE

Exercise can improve your asthma and protect you from this nation's number-one killer—heart disease. Regular exercise, especially aerobic exercise, strengthens your heart and lungs, adding healthy, active years to your life. Besides lowering your cholesterol and protecting you from heart disease, a healthy diet coupled with regular exercise reduces your risk of cancer, diabetes, hypertension, and a slew of other illnesses. Exercise helps you sleep better, increases energy levels, and boosts your immune system. Exercise will make you look better naked and improve your sex life. If you have diabetes, hypertension, depression, fibromyalgia, or virtually any other chronic medical problem, exercise can make your condition more manageable.

Even more important, exercise will make you feel great about yourself. As soon as you start to exercise and eat right, as soon as you make a commitment to healthy living, something magical happens: you take control of your life. By living healthily, you say to the world, "I am the master of my fate. I have control and this is my responsibility." We need this attitude both to beat asthma and to be successful in everything we do.

If you think asthma and exercise don't mix, take into consideration that there are many professional athletes with asthma. In fact, asthma (especially exercise-induced asthma or EIA) is actually more common in athletes. One study from Oslo, Norway, found that 10 percent of Norwegian elite athletes were asthmatic compared to 6.9 percent of the general population.[1] It is estimated that 4 to 15 percent of Summer Olympics athletes have asthma or use asthma medications.[2] According to one study, "the risk of asthma is especially increased among competitive swimmers, of which 36 percent to 79 percent show bronchial hyperresponsiveness."[3] One interesting study from the US Army Research Institute of Environmental Medicine examined the impact of EIA on army recruits and their ability to perform the Army Physical Fitness Test (APFT). The authors concluded that EIA "did not hinder their physical performance" and found that there was not a significant difference between the APFT scores of those with EIA and those without.[4]

Hyperventilation probably plays a leading role in the increased incidence of asthma in athletes. It is thought that in winter, hyperventilation exposes the athlete's lungs to tremendous volumes of cold, dry air, while in the summer, hyperventilation results in increased exposure to pollen and air pollution—all of which can trigger asthma.

Personally, I play harder and longer simply because I refuse to let asthma get me down. This is the same approach I want you to take toward exercise and asthma. Many asthmatics don't realize that it's OK to exercise. The common but mistaken belief that exercise is harmful or dangerous to people with asthma explains why many asthmatics are not fit. The truth is that asthma and exercise were meant for each other.

The Benefits of Exercise

There is an extensive body of literature documenting the health benefits of exercise and how it can help asthma. According to a study in the *Journal of Sports Medicine and Physical Fitness,* "there is substantial evidence that exercise training increases exercise performance and fitness in asthmatics."[5] In asthmatics, heart and lung function improve and medication use declines with exercise.

One study from Brazil examined the effect of aerobic exercise on forty-two children with moderate to severe asthma. As expected, exercise capacity improved and there was a significant reduction in the daily use of both inhaled and oral steroids.[6]

A Swedish study examined the impact of a ten-week exercise program on thirty-two asthmatics and found that "asthma symptoms declined during the rehabilitation period and the subjects needed less acute asthma care after the rehabilitation." Cardiovascular condition improved dramatically and there were no asthma attacks in conjunction with the training sessions.[7]

Exercise can even benefit people with emphysema and severe asthma, as one Swiss study demonstrated. After thirty-six aerobic-exercise sessions, thirteen patients with emphysema and asthma reported decreased shortness of breath and improved quality of life. Prior to the study, participants were only able to walk an average of 401 meters in six minutes, compared to 551 meters after rehabilitation.[8]

Furthermore, there is evidence that the benefits of exercise for asthma are not short-lived. One study followed thirty-nine mild to moderate asthmatics for three years after they participated in an exercise program. The authors found a significant decrease in the number of emergency-room visits in the three years following the rehabilitation program. There was also a decrease in asthma symptoms in all patients; however, this decrease was significant only in those patients who continued to exercise one to two times weekly.[9] Clearly, there are a substantial number of studies documenting that exercise can help people with asthma. So, how should an asthmatic exercise?

Exercise: The Basics

There are three basic exercises that everyone, including asthmatics, should do regularly: aerobic exercise, anaerobic exercise, and stretching. Stretching is the "orphan" of exercise, since few people seem to do it. Stretching is nevertheless important to help prevent injury and is an integral part of many relaxation and breathing techniques, such as yoga, that can help asthmatics. While all three exercises are important, aerobic exercise is probably the most vital for asthmatics. Aerobic exercises like walking, swimming, biking, and running help train your heart and lungs to work as a team. Aerobic exercise will also help your asthma and add healthy, active years to your life.

Aerobic Exercise

The type of aerobic exercise you choose depends on your level of physical fitness, personality, and asthma severity. If you've been a dedicated couch potato, start by walking for thirty minutes every day. You can walk in your neighborhood, the mall, or the woods. Where you walk depends on where you live and how comfortable you are with walking. If you're in good shape and otherwise healthy, you can walk anywhere. If you have several medical conditions and haven't walked by yourself for some time, walk where other people are present, like the mall. After two weeks of daily walking, increase your walk to an hour every day. As the weeks pass, increase the pace of your walk and include some hills for extra exercise. To make sure you're getting a good workout, you should be breathing a little harder and faster than normal, but not running out of breath or having to stop and rest.

Also, remember to stay hydrated during exercise. If you're exercising correctly, chances are you've worked up a sweat. Replacing water lost during exercise is especially important for asthmatics to prevent heat exhaustion and dehydration. Dehydration poses unique dangers for asthmatics, because the less water you have in your body, the thicker the mucus in your lungs. Thick mucus is one of the characteristics of an asthma attack. There is also evidence that dehydration may cause edema and bronchoconstriction in the lungs.

The best replacement fluid is good old-fashioned water. Those expensive "sports" drinks can actually promote dehydration by shifting water to your stomach to digest their sweeteners and electrolytes. What can happen is that you become increasingly dehydrated as your stomach tries to dilute the concentrated drink. For an asthmatic who is exercising, this fluid shift can rob the lungs of precious water that is needed to keep bronchial secretions thin. So, during exercise, take frequent but small sips of water to stay hydrated. Salt and electrolyte replacement is usually only needed by heavily perspiring athletes.

After a couple of months of dedicated walking, try biking, swimming, or joining an aerobics class. Once again, the type of activity you choose depends on your fitness level, personality, and where you live. If you live in a large city, biking may not be a realistic option; you might consider joining a gym, where you can swim or take an aerobics class. Gyms are also useful during air-quality alert days, when it may be dangerous for an asthmatic to exercise outdoors. Aerobics classes come in all shapes and sizes, so you should have no problem finding a class right for you. Since swimming, biking, and aerobics tend to be more intense than walking, you won't have to do them as often to stay in shape; 30–45 minutes every other day should be adequate.

With aerobic exercise, try to mix things up. If you perform the same exercise every day, your body will adapt and you won't get an effective workout. So, run one day, pound the stair-climbing machine the next, rest one day, then bike the next day—cross-training is great for your body.

With exercise, your mantra should be "Go slow and work my way up." For moderate-level aerobic exercise, you want to be breathing a little faster than you would while walking. Don't be embarrassed to rest if you need to, as it's better to gradually develop aerobic strength rather than overwork and potentially injure your body. My aversion to counting calories spills over into calculating heart rates. There are formulas for calculating target aerobic heart rate, which for most people are unnecessary. When exercising, pay attention to what your body tells you. You know you're getting a good workout if you're breathing fast but can still carry on a conversation. If you can't catch your breath or complete a sentence, you're exercising too hard and need to slow down. Unless you're in excellent, competitive-level shape, leave the heart-pounding, body-bashing stuff to the athletes.

For asthmatics who want to stay fit and do not intend to engage in high-intensity sports, I recommend sticking to moderate aerobic exercise. Moderate-level aerobic exercise offers similar health benefits as high-intensity aerobics without the risk of injury. If you begin to experience asthma symptoms while exercising, it's important to stop exercising immediately and treat the symptoms. Some asthmatics try to exercise through an asthma attack, a potentially dangerous practice that can lead to serious trouble.

Anaerobic Exercise

For most people, anaerobic exercise means weight lifting. Offering important health benefits, pumping iron will not only give you the strength necessary for aerobic exercise, but will also cause your body to preserve muscle mass. Preserving muscle mass becomes increasingly critical as we age, since our bodies normally replace muscle with fat. By lifting, you prevent this natural decline in muscle mass and protect yourself against conditions like diabetes. Because muscle consumes more sugar than fat, muscular people have a lower risk of diabetes than those who are obese.

The main reason to pump iron, however, is that the more muscle you have, the more you'll be able to run, walk, bike, or take part in whatever activity you choose. The good news is you don't have to look like a bodybuilder or bench press 300 pounds to benefit from weight training. Like aerobic exercise, weight lifting comes in all shapes and sizes. How much weight you lift depends on your fitness level and what you're trying to accomplish. I recommend starting with light weights and working your way up to moderate weights, leaving the heavy stuff for the bodybuilders.

"Light weights" means different things to different people and what is light for an eighteen-year-old is probably dangerous for an eighty-year-old. How much weight you start with is going to involve some trial and error. Ideally, you should feel resistance when lifting, with the weight neither too easy nor too hard to lift. You should not feel pain; if you feel pain, stop lifting immediately, rest a minute, and then resume lifting with a lighter weight.

If you're a true beginner, I recommend starting with five to twenty pounds for arm, chest, and shoulder exercises, and twenty to seventy pounds for leg exercises. There are many excellent books on weight lifting that can show you the basic exercises. While quality exercise equipment for home use is available, it can be expensive. Since all the machinery needed to perform multiple exercises can be found in most gyms, the gym is probably the best choice for beginners. There's also a safety issue: if you injure yourself, it helps to have other people around, rather than being home alone.

I strongly recommend that, if you're new to weight lifting, you join a gym and enlist the services of a personal trainer. This may seem expensive at first; however, a personal trainer knows which exercises and weight loads are right for you and will teach you how to lift correctly and safely. Once you've learned how to lift properly, you can go it alone. At the gym, you can also interact with like-minded individuals, supporting one another and learning from one another's successes and mistakes. As usual, always check with your doctor before starting an anaerobic or aerobic exercise program.

Remember, weight lifting is for everyone. Even people with severe medical conditions and disabilities can benefit from a properly tailored weight-lifting program. Multiple studies have found that regular aerobic and anaerobic exercise adds healthy years to one's life and can help prevent and ameliorate medical problems like diabetes and high blood pressure. Exercise is especially beneficial for individuals with chronic pain problems like rheumatoid arthritis or fibromyalgia, as several studies have demonstrated that people experience less pain when they exercise regularly.

Stretching: The Orphan of Exercise

Stretching is the orphan of exercise—everybody talks about it, but few do it. Stretching is nonetheless critical and an important part of your exercise regimen. The older we get, the more brittle we become and the more likely we are to be injured, especially during exercise. Stretching keeps your ligaments, tendons, and muscles strong and flexible. The stronger your muscles, the better your performance, whether you're playing football or casting a fly into your favorite stream. The same goes for flexibility: the more flexible you are, the better your performance and the less risk of injury.

Some say stretching is best done before exercising, while others say afterward is better. The available books on exercise will only add to your confusion about how, when, and why to stretch. Many people find stretching boring and don't do it at all. Fortunately, there are ways to make stretching more interesting. For instance, yoga is one of the best all-around exercises you can do, and I say this from personal experience. Yoga combines strength, flexibility, and balance—all essential to athletic performance. For instance, soon after I started doing yoga, my skiing skills zoomed up several notches. For those of you who think yoga is not really exercise, try sitting "Indian style" with one hand between your legs pressed firmly to the floor and lift yourself off the ground. No easy feat! Yoga comes in many different forms to suit every need; whether you're an Olympic athlete or a paraplegic, yoga has something to offer you.

Perhaps most important for asthmatics, yoga will teach you how to breathe. You may be thinking, "Teach me how to breathe? Hey! I've been breathing all my life." However, there is good breathing and bad breathing. By teaching proper diaphragmatic breathing techniques, yoga has helped many asthmatics lead better lives. In fact, as you will read in Chapter 9, dysfunctional breathing is *the* problem for many asthmatics, and breathing therapy can help them control their symptoms.

There is also a powerful mind-body connection that operates to different degrees in asthmatics. Asthma is frequently both a medical and a psychological problem. This does not mean that your asthma is all in your head, but rather that what goes on in your head has a lot to do with what goes on in your lungs. In this stressful world, asthmatics must learn to relax, a lesson that may prove difficult for many of us. With yoga, not only will you be perfecting your balance, flexibility, and strength, you'll also be helping your lungs by relieving stress and soothing your soul. I recommend 15–30 minutes of yoga before exercise.

If you're stressed out, try some peace and quiet with yoga or Tai Chi. Some of you may want more intensity: karate, judo, and kickboxing emphasize the same essentials as yoga, but from a different perspective. If you want to "sweat out" your stress, or build up your confidence in handling stressful situations, then one of these martial arts may be what you're looking for. Excellent books and videos can show you the moves, or you can hire a private instructor or take a group class. How you learn depends on how much you're willing to spend and on your unique personality. My advice is to just do it!

Asthma and the Athlete

If you like to ski, climb, mountain bike, or engage in any other strenuous activity, working your body hard is not a bad idea, as long as you're an otherwise healthy, well-conditioned asthmatic. In other words, asthma is no excuse for athletic mediocrity. Just ask track-and-field star Jackie Joyner-Kersee or swimmer Amy Van Dyken or Washington Redskins fullback Donnell Bennett—all asthmatics.

Before you join the local rugby team, make sure you've been performing mid- to high-level aerobic exercise, along with some weight training and stretching thrown in for good measure. Don't just roll out of bed one morning and decide that, after ten years of sitting in front of the TV, you're going to run marathons. This is not only a good way to get hurt, but you actually risk your life. If you've been exercising regularly, your asthma is under control, and you have no other medical problems that would stop you from strenuous exercise, then there's no reason why you shouldn't push yourself to the next level. Of course, it's always a good idea to talk to your doctor before embarking on an exercise program, especially one in which you intend to push your body hard.

Exercise-Induced Asthma

One of the potential problems asthmatics encounter during exercise is exercise-induced asthma (EIA). As a rule, the harder and faster you breathe, the greater your risk of EIA. EIA feels just like regular asthma except that the symptoms usually occur several minutes after you stop exercising. Preventing EIA is easy: Take two puffs of a beta-agonist, such as albuterol, fifteen minutes before exercise. Cromolyn sodium is another medication used to prevent EIA (taken as two puffs within an hour of exercise). If you'd rather avoid medications, there are several natural remedies that can help prevent EIA, such as vitamin C (see Chapter 7).

Breathing hard and fast is an unavoidable and healthy part of strenuous exercise. What really promotes EIA is not how hard or fast you breathe but the temperature and humidity of the air you're breathing. The lower the temperature and humidity, the greater the risk of EIA. This is why so many asthmatics have trouble in the winter, especially with outdoor sports. Don't despair, because the well-prepared asthmatic can exercise safely, even in the winter.

The lungs don't want air that is too cold or dry, forcing them to work extra hard to warm and humidify the air as it enters the body. This rapid exchange of heat and moisture is blamed for triggering bronchoconstriction and causing EIA. This is why smart asthmatics make sure they cover their mouth and nose with a fabric before venturing into the cold. Breathing through fabric causes the material to become warm and moist, thereby preheating and premoisturizing the air before it hits your lungs. This helps the lungs avoid radical shifts in temperature and humidity, thereby lowering the risk of EIA. The role of cold, dry air in EIA was shown in a study that examined the effect of inhaling humidified air at body temperature in asthmatics. According to this study, warming and humidifying the air virtually eliminated EIA.[10]

How you cover your mouth and nose depends on what you're doing. If you're going for a simple walk, a scarf works fine. If you're climbing mountains and plan to be in very cold weather for a long time, a balaclava (combination face mask, hat, and neck scarf) is probably best. Wool and fleece are the most winter-friendly fabrics, because they retain heat even when wet. Cotton is not recommended, as it tends to freeze and rob your body of heat when moist. This same technique works indoors if you happen to be very sensitive to exercise. The only potential problem with covering your face indoors is that you run the risk of overheating. During exercise, you lose a tremendous amount of heat from the lungs, neck, and head. Not allowing excess heat to escape can limit your performance and may even cause heat exhaustion. So, if you're going to cover your face indoors, use a small face mask that covers no more than your mouth and nose, and dress a bit lighter than usual to help prevent you from getting too hot.

If you've done all the right things but are still having EIA trouble, try moving your exercise indoors. For most asthmatics, this should help; however, there will be a small percentage of people who are very susceptible to EIA no matter what they do. For these individuals, I recommend swimming in an indoor, heated pool, one of the safest and best-tolerated exercises for asthmatics. Besides being in a warm and humid, lung-friendly environment, swimming is an exercise that anyone can do regardless of their fitness level. Swimming is one of the best all-around exercises, combining aerobic and anaerobic conditioning. You can swim as fast or as slow as you want, from a leisurely backstroke to a brisk butterfly. You don't even have to swim to exercise in a pool. Most fitness clubs offer a range of water aerobics classes that cater to everyone, from recovering couch potato Olympic hopeful. Even people with severe medical problems or disabilities can exercise safely in a pool.

Are there any sports in which asthmatics should not participate? The only sport I wouldn't recommend is scuba diving, because there is evidence that asthmatics and people with EIA are at greater risk of diving-related barotrauma, a type of lung injury caused by rapid changes in lung pressure.

OBESITY AND ASTHMA

Seemingly everywhere you look, there's a book, magazine, or advertisement on weight loss. In the United States, almost 20 percent of the population is medically obese. Staying slim is about more than just good looks. Obesity is one of the most devastating illnesses known, because it contributes to a number of medical conditions, such as diabetes, hypertension, heart disease, lung disease, arthritis, and depression. There is also active research on the association between asthma and obesity. One study from the University of Ottawa, in Canada, examined 9,149 adults and found that obese women, but not men, had almost twice the risk of asthma.[11] Another prospective, ten-year study of 4,547 adults also found that obesity increased asthma risk in women, but not in men.[12] Finally, a survey of 7,109 adults, conducted by the Brigham and Women's Hospital in Boston, found that "both underweight and overweight are associated with increased risk of asthma" in women.[13] Why obesity does not clearly increase the risk of asthma in men is a question presently undergoing investigation.

Besides reducing your risk of asthma, there are clearly other compelling, health-related reasons to maintain an ideal weight. Once again, obesity dramatically increases your risk of diabetes, heart disease, hypertension, and arthritis. As mentioned previously, don't fixate on weight loss;

rather, your efforts should remain focused on healthy living. If you exercise and eat right, you will be amazed at how quickly you lose weight and how much better you feel physically and mentally. Eating right and exercising are two parts of the healthy-living triad. The third part is getting enough sleep.

ASTHMA AND SLEEP

I probably don't need to tell you that asthma and sleep are not friends. Sleep is, however, one of our most important bodily functions and the foundation on which our health rests. Sleep deprivation weakens the immune system, limits the ability to concentrate and remember, and is a major contributor to automobile accidents. One study from the University of Oxford found that "children with asthma [had] significantly more disturbed sleep [and] performed less well on some tests of memory and concentration."[14] Sleeping is a serious business.

So how does an asthmatic get a good night's sleep? The first step is to understand that sleep is, in part, a learned behavior. The best sleepers never need an alarm clock and have trained their bodies to hit the sack and arise every day at the same time. We all have an internal clock that tells us when to sleep and when to wake up. Training this clock and habituating sleep are the keys to sound slumber. If you follow these seven "rules," you'll establish a healthy routine and sleep like a baby.

Rule 1: Wake Up at the Same Time Every Day

By waking up at the same time every day, you tell your internal clock, "This is the time I need to get up." When I say "every day," I mean religiously waking up at the same time every weekday and on the weekend. Waking up late resets your internal clock, which is why people who sleep in on weekends have a terrible time getting up Monday morning.

Rule 2: Go to Bed Only When Tired

By going to bed only when you are tired, you're more likely to fall asleep quickly with a minimum of tossing and turning. In fact, tossing and turning is one of the worst things you can do in bed. If you can't fall asleep after twenty minutes, get up and do something relaxing until you're tired and ready to return to bed. This same advice applies to when you wake up in the middle of the night and can't get back to sleep.

Rule 3: No Daytime Naps

We're training your body and internal clock to associate the bed with a full night's sleep. Daytime naps fragment and reduce your overall sleep quality by telling your body it's OK to be tired and fall asleep during the day. If you have an irresistible urge to nap, I suggest doing something stimulating like exercise or showering. The same advice applies to night-shift workers: Only go to bed when you're ready to commit yourself to six to ten hours of sleep.

Rule 4: The Bedroom Is for Sleep and Sex Only

Make your bedroom a refuge from the troubles and stresses of life, a haven of peace and relaxation. This means no TV, work, or food in the bedroom. Train your body and mind to associate the bedroom and the bed with sleep and sex only. Also, keep your bedroom as quiet and dark as possible, since lights and noise fragment sleep.

Rule 5: Don't Be a Clock-Watcher

When you hit the sack, make sure your alarm clock is set and turned away from you so you can't roll over at three in the morning and say, "Oh no, it's three in the morning and I'm still awake!" By checking your clock, you'll realize how late it is and start calculating how many hours you can sleep. Thus begins a vicious cycle of clock-watching and worrying that will never allow you to rest comfortably. Losing a night's sleep is no big deal, so stop worrying about the time.

Rule 6: No Alcohol, Caffeine, Exercise, or Heavy Meals Before Bed

Alcohol may help you fall asleep but will ultimately corrupt your sleep quality. Caffeine, a stimulant, can prevent you from falling asleep. If you can't live without caffeine, get your fix in the morning. Also, avoid heavy meals three to four hours before bed. Having a full stomach while laying flat increases your risk of gastroesophageal reflux, a major contributor to GERD and asthma that can ruin a good night's sleep. It's OK to eat a light snack before bed, just don't make it a five-course meal. Avoid sweet snacks before bedtime, since sugar is a stimulant and, like caffeine, can prevent you from falling asleep. Finally, do not exercise during the four to five hours prior to bedtime, as the stimulating effects of exercise may keep you awake.

Rule 7: Make Bedtime a Habit

Always do something relaxing before bed, such as reading a book or taking a warm bath. Don't take a shower before bed, since showers tend to stimulate rather than relax. By performing the same relaxing activity an hour prior to bedtime, you clear your mind of everyday concerns and tell your body that bedtime is near. Don't go to bed immediately after returning home from a hard day's work, as you'll only spend half the night tossing and turning. Take an hour and do something nice to forget the day's stress.

Perhaps the most important thing you can do to get a good night's sleep is to relax. If you worry about falling asleep, you virtually guarantee a night of tossing, turning, and clock-watching. If you follow these rules, you may be sleepy and uncomfortable for a week or two as your body adjusts, but then you'll establish a healthy sleep cycle and get the sleep you need.

How much sleep do you need? Everybody is different with respect to how much sleep they need. Some people live on five hours a night, others need ten. On average, people need six to ten hours of sleep a night. Don't worry about how much sleep you get; rather, concentrate on establishing healthy sleep habits and your body will let you know how much sleep it wants.

ELIMINATING BAD HABITS: TOBACCO, ALCOHOL, AND DRUGS

One of the tragic lessons we learned in Chapter 1 is that most asthma deaths are preventable. What is particularly notable is the large number of people who have died from asthma who were abusing tobacco, alcohol, or drugs at the time of death. If you don't smoke or abuse drugs and drink only in moderation, you have a much better prospect of living a long life with asthma. If, however, you have any of these bad habits, not only are you more likely to die from asthma, but you also risk developing emphysema, cancer, and cirrhosis of the liver. These habits are literally killers of asthmatics, so I urge you to give them up now.

Smoking

Need I tell you that smoking is bad for your asthma? I understand the smoking problem. Nicotine is a powerful drug that some say is more addictive than cocaine. From the age of thirteen to twenty-three, I smoked a pack of cigarettes a day, and quitting was not easy. Even ten years after quitting I had cravings and now, almost two decades later, I still dream about smoking. An exhaustive discussion on how to quit is beyond the scope of this book; however, I want you to understand what smoking does to your lungs and follow it up with some advice on how to quit.

Tobacco smoke has over 4,000 different compounds, forty of which cause cancer in humans. Of all the oxidant stressors, smoking is probably the most devastating. The free radicals generated by tobacco decimate vitamins C and E, the lung's chief antioxidants. Once reserves of vitamins C and E are depleted, your lungs are prone to oxidative damage. Also, immunoglobulin E (IgE) and eosinophils are present in higher-than-normal levels in smokers and the children of smokers. Children of smokers have a higher incidence of lung disease, asthma, childhood illnesses, and hospitalizations. Even more disturbing, the asthma seen in the children of smokers tends to be worse than the asthma found in children from smoke-free homes. Smokers also have increased airway reactivity that becomes worse with time. What this translates into for asthmatics is, the more you smoke, the worse your asthma.

If you decide to quit smoking, the best advice I can offer is to let everyone know you're quitting and never smoke the same brand of cigarette twice. If you announce your intention to quit and then resume smoking, you let yourself and everyone you know down, a powerful incentive for sticking with your resolution to quit. Switching brands each time you buy cigarettes takes some of the pleasure out of smoking. Tobacco abuse is a double-edged sword: you not only get hooked on nicotine but also develop a taste for a particular brand of cigarette. By choosing a different brand each time you buy cigarettes, you increase your chances of quitting.

Don't be discouraged if at first you fail. The average smoker tries to quit many times before succeeding. Even after you quit, the battle is only half over, because for several years you'll be constantly tempted to light up. To increase your chances of success, establish an alliance with a trusted healthcare professional who can offer you a variety of pharmacological or natural remedies to aid your recovery. Once you have stopped smoking, try to avoid breathing in second-hand smoke. Second-hand smoke is bad for your health and provides a tempting reminder to your brain of the nicotine it craves. Staying away from tobacco smoke will keep your lungs honest.

If you have the misfortune of living with a smoker, sit down and explain to this person what their smoking is doing to your health and lungs. If they can't quit, then they will have to smoke outside. The same goes for company, friends, relatives, or anyone who wants to smoke in your home. Guard your home like a mother bear protects her cubs and insist that your abode remain a smoke-free environment. If you cannot guarantee a smoke-free environment, then read Chapter 6 to learn how to purify your home's air.

Alcohol and Illegal Drugs

Given the high percentage of people who die from asthma while abusing drugs or alcohol, it is clear that alcohol and drug abuse don't mix with asthma. I have no objection to a moderate amount of alcohol every now and then. There are recognized health benefits associated with moderate alcohol use, especially wine. In fact, according to a study from King's College in London on the dietary habits of 9,709 individuals, red wine intake was negatively associated with asthma severity due to the protective effects of flavonoids contained in the wine.[15] Weighing against the benefits of moderate alcohol use is the fact that sulfites, commonly used as a preservative in alcoholic beverages, are toxic to the lungs and can trigger asthma attacks in sensitized individuals. However, for the vast majority of people, especially asthmatics, it's heavy drinking that causes trouble. So, if you have a glass of wine with your evening meal, you should be OK as long as you limit yourself to one drink a day. If you think you may have an alcohol problem, I strongly suggest you seek profession help.

Drug abuse is totally incompatible with asthma. Not only do illegal drugs take a devastating toll on your body, but a significant percentage of people who died from asthma have been subsequently found to have recently used illegal drugs.

ADDITIONAL HEALTHY-LIVING TIPS

It is especially important for asthmatics to protect themselves from catching those nasty colds that cause so much trouble. By eating, exercising, and sleeping right, you strengthen your immune system to fight viral invaders. Like it or not, viruses are everywhere and they can't be avoided. The good news is that you can avoid most viral infections with a few simple steps.

Frequent hand washing is the best defense against infection. Infections usually begin in one of two ways: you either inhale germs from the air or pick up the germs on your hands and then touch your face. The bacteria then enter your body through the nose, mouth, or eyes, and the infection gets under way. This is why it's so important to wash your hands several times a day and keep them away from your face, especially after using the bathroom or touching other people, before eating, or after coming into contact with someone who has a cold. A simple habit like regular hand washing goes a long way toward keeping you and your asthma trouble-free.

My other suggestion is that you try to avoid people who are sick. This may be easier said than done, especially if you have children; however, when logistically and socially possible, try to avoid people with colds. If your significant other or spouse is sick, perhaps it's not a bad idea to sleep in a spare bedroom or couch for few nights. Kissing sick people is obviously not a good idea. If you find yourself in the company of someone who is ill, wash your hands immediately after the encounter and try not to let them touch you. Admittedly, this may seem a bit cold and impersonal; however, after explaining to your friends the trouble that the common cold can cause an asthmatic, they should understand.

chapter 6

Home Decorating for the Asthmatic

In the last several years, a growing body of scientific evidence has indicated that the air within homes and other buildings can be more seriously polluted than the outdoor air in even the largest and most industrialized cities. Other research indicated that people spend approximately 90 percent of their time indoors.[1]

—US ENVIRONMENTAL PROTECTION AGENCY

The most predictable health benefit will be achieved by eliminating the source of the allergen from the home—be it a pet or a heavily mite-infested sofa—or by environmental control measures designed to decrease the exposure of mite allergen.[2]

—NATIONAL JEWISH CENTER FOR IMMUNOLOGY AND RESPIRATORY MEDICINE

HOME, SWEET HOME! Unfortunately, home may not be so sweet if you have asthma; your home may be the reason you have asthma. How can this be? Because your home is also an abode for dust, bugs, and toxins that can make your lungs miserable. Topping the list of home-environment asthma triggers are cat and dog dander, cockroach droppings, and dust mites. Also on the list are cooking smells, laundry detergents, soaps, perfumes, gardens, pesticides, tobacco smoke, hobby supplies, and many others.

As I mentioned briefly in Chapter 1, indoor air pollution is emerging as a major factor in the asthma epidemic. Since the energy crisis of the 1970s, new energy-efficient homes are frequently built airtight. While this is a smart idea for conserving energy, it also means these homes are especially good at keeping stale, polluted air inside the house. Add to this the prevalence of central heating and air-conditioning, synthetic chemical-laden building materials, and wall-to-wall carpeting—it's no surprise that indoor air is frequently more polluted than outdoor air.

Hippocrates first observed the relationship between asthma and the "prevailing winds." Let's face it, for most asthmatics it's something in the air that's causing the problem. Even for idiopathic asthmatics, it is likely that they too are reacting to something airborne, but we just haven't figured out the trigger yet.

According to the Environmental Protection Agency (EPA), air pollution is divided into three broad categories: particulate matter, gaseous pollutants, and radon. Particulate matter includes mites, dander, dust, molds, and pollen. Gaseous pollution can emanate from cleaning agents, deodorants, dyes, or the burning of fuels (such as gas, oil, wood, tobacco, car exhaust). Second-hand tobacco smoke is especially dangerous for asthmatics, harming the lungs with toxic oxidants. You may also be surprised to learn that many gaseous pollutants originate from building materials and furniture, especially particleboard. Radon comes from natural materials, such as soil and rock, but can also emerge from mineral-based building materials. These pollutants have the potential to cause numerous medical problems, including allergies, asthma, and cancer. Conversely, cleaning up or eliminating these sources of pollution can bring a great deal of relief to asthmatics.

HOW TO PROTECT YOUR LUNGS

In a world filled with toxins, how can you best protect your lungs? You can always try holding your breath, but that only goes so far. The best protection, without question, is to remove the offending agent; this is known as "source control." Source control has a long history, dating back to the sixteenth century, when Italian physician Girolamo Cardano recommended that the Archbishop of St. Andrews get rid of his feather bedding. It was subsequently reported that the Archbishop had a "miraculous" recovery from his symptoms.

Later in this chapter, we'll go from room to room and identify the most common asthma triggers in each and learn how to eliminate them. During this process, as you discover your unique asthma triggers, you'll need to decide if you can live without a particular trigger. For some triggers, this may be as simple as asking a family member not to buy a particular perfume or cologne. Other triggers may be a bit more complicated, like switching from a gas to an electric stove.

While source control will always remain the gold standard for asthma prevention, removing some irritants, such as pollen and formaldehyde, may be impractical or impossible. For instance, it's easy to switch from scented to unscented laundry detergent, but not so easy to move the family from pollen-packed Fresno, California, to the desert. How do you manage those triggers for which source control is not practical? By ventilating and purifying the air you breathe.

VENTILATION: OPEN THE WINDOW

Your grandmother probably used to say, "Open the window and let the fresh air in!" She was onto something—ventilation. Unless you live in a polluted city or next to a petrochemical plant, chances are that the air outside your home is cleaner than the air inside it. So, let the bad air out and the good air in. Every day, open your home's windows, and turn on the bathroom and kitchen exhaust fans, to exchange "dirty" inside air for "clean" outdoor air. After you have ventilated your home for ten to thirty minutes, you can then shut your windows and start your air-cleaning system (discussed below). You should also ventilate your home while vacuuming, cooking, or painting—any activity that potentially produces particulate or gaseous pollution. If possible, take asthma-dangerous activities like sanding or working with airplane glue outdoors.

With the advent of airtight, energy-efficient homes and offices, ventilation has become an increasingly sophisticated business. Ventilating your home, however, can be expensive if you must reheat or cool the exchanged air. Consider installing energy-efficient ventilation systems that can be used in the winter without losing much heat. Called "air-to-air heat exchangers" or "heat recovery ventilators," they may be worth the cost for some asthmatics. For more information on air-to-air heat exchangers, contact:

Renewable Energy Inquiry and Referral Service (CAREIRS)
PO Box 3048
Merrifield, VA 22116
Website: www.p2000.umich.edu/appendix.html

Don't ventilate your home when there are air-quality alerts; rather, let your air-conditioning or cleaning system do the dirty work, particularly if the weather is hot or muggy. Air conditioners are great for asthmatics;

there is evidence that air-conditioning may be more effective than air cleaners or purifiers for removing pollutants. During warm summer months, air-conditioning is often superior to air cleaning simply because air conditioners recirculate indoor air and keep humidity levels low, thereby creating a hostile environment for mold growth. Speaking of mold, if you're sensitive to pollen or mold, keep your windows closed during days when pollen or mold counts are high. Most people, even city dwellers, have decent outdoor air and can ventilate their homes or apartments safely for the greater part of the year. If you have any concerns about air pollution, call the local health department and ask for a daily air-quality report.

Besides opening windows, use your kitchen and bathroom exhaust fans liberally to remove pollutants that often accumulate in these areas. Some asthmatics take air exchange a step further by ventilating their attics and crawlspaces, thereby keeping their home's humidity level below 50 percent and inhibiting mold growth. Finally, make sure your clothes dryer is ventilated to the outside, not the inside, of your house.

AIR CLEANERS AND PURIFIERS

When coupled with source control, aggressive ventilation is probably all that many asthmatics will ever need. If, however, you have seasonal allergic asthma or are sensitive to outdoor air pollution, there may be irritants in the "good" outdoor air that can trigger your asthma. This is where air cleaners and purifiers can be beneficial. Air cleaners come in all shapes and sizes, but there are three basic types: mechanical air filters, electronic air filters, and ionizers. Likewise, air cleaners perform three basic functions: filtering particulate matter, removing gaseous pollution, and circulating air. Air cleaning is a complicated subject, so let's first look at filtering particulate pollution.

Filtering Particulate Pollution

It is important to remove both large particles that cause allergic reactions and small respirable particles that can find their way deep inside the lung and cause damage. Particle filters range from the boxed filter on your furnace to high-tech, asthma-friendly High Energy Particulate Air (HEPA) filters, which trap almost all airborne contaminants.

Mechanical Air Filters

Mechanical filters used to be packed with fiberglass or some other fine fiber that was treated with a "sticky" substance to help trap particles and boost efficiency. The filter would be either flat or pleated, with the pleats dramatically increasing surface area. As filtering technology improved, these simple fiber filters were given an electrostatic charge that could trap even smaller airborne particles. These basic fiber-based mechanical filters are still made and are commonly found at the local hardware store. In fact, if you look at your furnace or air-conditioning intake vent, you'll probably see one of these mechanical filters. Despite the technological innovations, fiber-based filters still only trap the largest particles; they simply don't cut it when it comes to asthma.

Filter technology has fortunately continued to mature, and there are filters specially designed for people with allergies and asthma. To be designated a HEPA filter, these state-of-the-art air filters must have a minimum collection efficiency of 99.97 percent. If you have allergic asthma or suspect your lungs are bothered by particulate pollution, a HEPA filter can be your best friend.

Electronic Air Cleaners

HEPA filters represent the cutting-edge in mechanical air filtration and will probably remain an industry standard for years to come. However, "electronic precipitators" or electronic air cleaners are an emerging technological innovation. Using less electricity and operating noiselessly, electronic precipitators have found a place in bedrooms across America. Electronic air cleaners employ a charged filter to collect particles. Many manufacturers add ionizers to their units that place a charge on airborne particles before they enter the system, thereby making these particles more "sticky" and improving collection efficacy. Electronic air cleaners can be used alone or combined with a HEPA filter. A potential drawback to electronic air cleaners is that they can lose efficiency if not properly maintained. Another problem with electronic precipitators is that some models produce ozone, a gas that is especially troublesome to some asthmatics.

Though HEPA filters have an established track record, you may want to consider the new HEPA/electronic precipitator hybrids, while avoiding units that produce ozone. I suspect that as technology improves, electronic precipitators may emerge as a superior air-purifying product.

Ionizers

Ionizers place an electric charge on particulate pollutants so they will stick to an oppositely charged surface. This means that unless the ionizer is combined with a collection filter, the charged particles will end up sticking to anything: floors, drapes, furniture, and even people. In my opinion, ionizers don't clean the air, they just stick pollution elsewhere. Unless it comes with a collection device, don't buy an ionizer.

Ozone Generators

Some manufacturers add ozone generators to their air cleaners, claiming that ozone "freshens" and "cleans" the air. Ozone, however, is a reactive oxygen species that asthmatics clearly should avoid. According to the EPA, ozone can be unhealthy with little potential to remove indoor air contaminants.[3] Ozone generators are dangerous to your health and simply don't work.

Air Fresheners

My advice on scented "air fresheners" is to throw them out. Scented air fresheners only mask one odor with another and do absolutely nothing to improve air quality. Many asthmatics, including myself, are driven nuts by the smell of air fresheners.

Filtering Gaseous and Chemical Pollution

Particles are only part of the air-pollution problem. Quality air purifiers remove both particulate matter and gaseous and chemical pollution, a process called "sorption." Without question, asthmatics need air cleaners that perform both functions well. Most sorption systems use a sorbent, such as activated carbon, to suck up chemical and gas fumes. Like mechanical air filters, sorption systems receive an efficiency rating based on the amount of chemical and/or gas absorbed. Sorbents do not last forever and, like particulate air filters, the more material they absorb, the less efficient they become, so you have to periodically replace the sorbent.

Activated carbon is a common sorbent that works well even in humid environments. Carbon is also an excellent odor absorber; however, just because you can't smell anything doesn't mean the toxin is gone. Carbon filters may remove the smell, but the toxin can still be present at imperceptible levels and thereby impact your health. Carbon filters also tend to get saturated quickly, necessitating frequent replacement. Filter saturation not only reduces efficiency but also may cause the filter to reemit chemicals into the environment. Once again, the best way to deal with noxious fumes is source control; if you remove the source of the irritant, you won't have to worry about absorbing it.

If source control is impractical or not possible, activated carbon is your best, albeit imperfect, choice. Activated carbon is one of several sorbents, some of which are designed for specific chemicals like formaldehyde. As a rule, specialized sorbents outperform activated carbon; however, unless you have identified a specific chemical substance to which you are sensitive, most asthmatics do well using an activated carbon filter. No matter what type of filter you use, always follow the manufacturer's recommendations regarding replacement.

Evaluating Air Cleaners

What makes an excellent portable air cleaner? Two words: efficiency and ventilation. Efficiency relates to the percentage of airborne contaminants removed by the filter. For asthma sufferers, HEPA filters are most efficient, since they trap nearly all airborne contaminants. The second and equally critical feature is ventilating power—how much air the unit can filter within a certain period of time, usually expressed as cubic feet per minute. Ventilating power is important because you want to clean all the room's air within a reasonable time frame. Most units are rated for a specific cubic volume of air, so all you need to know is your room's volume. For instance, if you're purchasing an air cleaner for the bedroom, calculate the volume of your bedroom and match this against the unit's rating. If your bedroom is 1,000 cubic feet, you need a purifier that is rated for a minimum of 1,000 cubic feet. To calculate cubic volume, multiply the room's length times the width times the height.

Related to ventilation is operating speed. Quality air cleaners can run at different speeds. How fast you decide to ventilate a room depends on what you're doing. A high speed should be used after vacuuming or cooking, when you want to filter the air rapidly. Lower speeds are usually reserved for day-to-day, continual air purifying.

Ideally, you want a highly efficient unit that can ventilate the target volume of air several times an hour. Manufacturers use fancy names like "clean air delivery rate," "atmospheric dust spot test," and "military standard 2823" to rate ventilating power. To evaluate these ratings, visit the EPA website: www.epa.gov/iaq/pubs/residair.html.

Size is also important when it comes to air cleaners. Table and desktop models are usually not as efficient or powerful as larger console models. If you don't want portable units clashing with your interior design, call your local Heating, Ventilating, and Air Conditioning (HVAC) specialist to discuss induct air-purifying systems, which are designed to service your entire home.

Air-Cleaner Shortcomings

While air purifiers sound like a great idea, they are really the products of last resort. The best defense against air pollution will always be source control and ventilation. If your home is jammed with flowering potted plants, perhaps it would be in your best interest to put those plants outside rather than buy an expensive air cleaner. Air cleaners can make a difference, but they are not perfect. They can lose efficiency as their filters, precipitators, or sorbents become saturated with pollutants. Equally concerning, as a filter captures more and more pollutants and becomes saturated, the filter itself may begin to deliver harmful gasses, odors, and particles into the air. This means you must pay meticulous attention to recommended maintenance and filter changes.

As for odors, while activated carbon removes many odors, most machines cannot remove every odor. Avoid air cleaners that "scent" the air, making it smell "fresh." Scenting only replaces one odor with another and does nothing to remove harmful fumes. Also, stay away from products that make ozone, a reactive gas known to trigger asthma. Finally, some asthmatics are sensitive to formaldehyde found in building materials like particleboard. Particleboard may be used in small appliances like air cleaners and should be avoided.

The limitations of air-cleaning technology were examined in 1997 by an ad hoc committee of air-cleaner manufacturers, who met at the request of the US Food and Drug Administration. According to the commission, "the data presently available are inadequate to establish the utility of these devices in the prevention and treatment of allergic respiratory disease." The committee went on to conclude that "air-cleaning devices should only be considered if symptoms remain severe despite other avoidance measures and there is reason to believe that a significant load of airborne allergens is present."[4] Likewise, studies in the scientific literature offer mixed results. One study on air filtration found that while there was a "trend" toward higher peak flows and a reduction in airborne pollutants, no difference in subjective symptoms or bronchial reactivity was demonstrated.[5] Bottom line: Source control and ventilation will do more to clean your air than any air cleaner; air cleaners are the refuge of last resort.

Let's examine in more detail why air cleaners are only a small part of the asthma solution. For an air cleaner to work, irritants must be airborne so they can enter the cleaning unit and be filtered. The problem is that most asthma triggers, like dander, are rarely airborne; they are usually trapped in the carpet, furniture, or bedding. These irritants travel into your airway when you disrupt them—such as by sitting on a piece of furniture, making the bed, or walking on or vacuuming the carpet—thereby causing them to become airborne. This is why experts recommend excluding carpeting, drapes, and other textiles from the homes of asthmatics and allergy sufferers. It is also the reason why source control is your best hope of relief; if you can eliminate an irritant at its source, you don't have to worry about that allergen getting into your bedding, carpeting, furniture, or lungs.

Information on Air Cleaners: A Resource List

Air cleaning technology is relatively new and, with the exception of self-imposed industry standards, there are no federal regulations regarding efficiency. In fact, industry standards only apply to particulate matter and at present there are no standards for gas or radon.

- For further information on air cleaners or industry standards, contact:
  Air-Conditioning & Refrigeration Institute (ARI)
  4301 North Fairfax Drive, Suite 425
  Arlington, VA 22203
  Phone: 703-524-8800 • Fax: 703-528-3816
  Website: www.ari.org

- The Association of Home Appliance Manufacturers (AHAM) rates air cleaners according to industry standards. This information is available on the Internet: www.cadr.org/cadr_flash.html. They have also published the *American National Standard Method for Measuring Performance of Portable Household Electric Cord-Connected Room Air Cleaners* (ANSI/AHAM AC-1-1988), which can be requested from:
  Association of Home Appliance Manufacturers
  1111 19th Street, NW, Suite 402
  Washington, DC 20036
  Phone: 202-872-5955 • Fax: 202-872-9354
  Website: www.aham.org

- The Environmental Protection Agency (EPA) has several excellent publications examining indoor air quality. The following is a partial list of those available on the Internet:
    - *The Inside Story: A Guide to Indoor Air Quality* EPA 402-K-93-007 (Washington, DC: US EPA, US CPSC, April 1995). Available on the EPA website: www.epa.gov/iaq/pubs/insidest.html.
    - *Indoor Air Facts No. 7—Residential Air Cleaners* EPA 20A-4-001 (Washington, DC: US EPA, February 1990). Available on the EPA website: www.epa.gov/iaq/pubs/airclean.html.
    - *Residential Air Cleaning Devices: A Summary of Available Information* EPA 400/1-90-002 (Washington, DC: US EPA, February 1990). Available on the EPA website: www.epa.gov/iaq/pubs/residair.html.
    - *Indoor Air Pollution: An Introduction for Health Professionals* US Government Printing Office Publication No. 1994-523-217/81322 (Washington, DC: The American Lung Association, US EPA, The Consumer Product Safety Commission, and The American Medical Association, 1994). Available on the EPA website: www.epa.gov/iaq/pubs/hpguide/html.

- You can also order documents directly from the EPA:

  US EPA
  National Center for Environmental Publications
  PO Box 42419
  Cincinnati, OH 45242
  Phone: 800-490-9198 • Fax: 513-489-8695
  Website: www.epa.gov/ncepihom

- If you don't have a computer or access to the Internet, you can get these publications by contacting:

  Superintendent of Documents
  US Government Printing Office (GPO)
  PO Box 371954
  Pittsburgh, PA 15250-7954
  Phone: 202-512-1800 • Fax: 202-512-2250

- Another excellent source of EPA information on indoor air quality can be found at:

  Indoor Air Quality Information Clearinghouse (IAQ INFO)

PO Box 37133
Washington, DC 20013-7133
Phone: 800-438-4318 • Fax: 703-356-5386
Website: www.epa.gov/iaq/iaqinfo.html

- Air pollution questions can also be answered by state agencies, which can be found through IAQ INFO. Many of the documents mentioned in this chapter can also be ordered through IAQ INFO.

Immediate Steps to Take for Cleaner Air

Look at your furnace or air-conditioning intake vent and locate the air filters—the same filters you probably haven't changed in some time. Don't be embarrassed, it took me over a year to change my air filters and I should know better. You can strike a blow against asthma today by changing every air filter you can find; look at your ceiling vents, furnace, and air conditioner. Check the owner's manual or call your service company to learn how often you need to change these filters. Ask the service representative or manufacturer if they sell special asthma- or allergy-friendly filters for their appliances.

Deciding on a HEPA filter with a quality gas and fume absorber in a rapidly ventilating unit should be easy. The hard part is deciding between acquiring portable/modular air cleaners or refitting your entire HVAC system with an induct filtration unit. While you can't control what happens to the air outside your house, you can control what happens to the air inside. If you have central air-conditioning or forced-air heat, there is ductwork that essentially monopolizes the air you breathe. Somewhere, probably on the ceiling, is an air-intake vent that sucks air into the HVAC system, which then spews it back into your home through a series of vents. Even if you don't have central air-conditioning or forced-air heat, your home may have some type of ventilation system.

A clean and efficient HVAC system can do wonders for asthma. Many people with asthma have trouble with "something" in the air and need to get it out of the air so it no longer irritates their lungs. The best way to rid that "something" from the air remains source control and ventilation. When source control and ventilation are impractical or impossible, such as with seasonal allergies, it's time to consider HVAC filtering systems. If you think an induct air-purifying system sounds right for you, call your local HVAC specialist to learn more.

Finally, your HVAC system has two ends: one for intake and one for output. Most homes have a single intake vent with multiple output vents. If you want to be meticulous, consider purchasing an electrostatic output vent filter to capture any contaminants your induct system may miss.

If you rarely use your furnace or air conditioner, or if you own an induct system but want extra help with trouble spots like the kitchen, consider a portable/modular air cleaner. As discussed previously, choose a portable air cleaner that uses a HEPA filter with a fume and odor sorbent in a unit that is rated for the room volume you want to clean. Pay attention to where you place your air purifier since location impacts efficiency. For example, to remove cooking fumes, place the unit's intake vent near the stove so the machine can suck up noxious fumes before they reach your lungs. But don't place the unit so close to the stove that it becomes a fire hazard. If your air cleaner is too hot to touch while cooking, it's probably too close to the stove. Finally, be careful not to block the unit's intake and output vents with furniture, walls, or appliances.

The nice part about portable air cleaners is that you turn them on and, with the exception of an occasional filter change, basically ignore them. Many people put their first unit in the bedroom, so it's important to buy a machine that runs quietly or is "noiseless." Usually, the quieter the machine, the more expensive it is, but a good night's sleep is worth the extra money. The bedroom is a logical place to start air purifying considering we spend a third of our lives in bed. Furthermore, the bedroom is one of the most hostile environments for asthmatics. How many HEPA units you use will depend on how aggressive you want to be; it's not unreasonable for some asthmatics to have a HEPA unit in every room.

One final note: Always change portable air filters outside, since old filters are loaded with contaminants that can be released back into the air with manipulation. The same advice applies to changing activated carbon filters and cleaning electrostatic precipitators. All used filters should be discarded in an outdoor trash container.

HUMIDITY

Why do some asthma and allergy sufferers flee to Arizona? It's the lack of humidity there. High humidity attracts dust mites and mold, both of which cause major problems for asthmatics because they dramatically increase the severity of asthma symptoms and reduce lung function in sensitized individuals. Keeping your home's humidity level between 30 and 50 percent can help you breathe. Air conditioners work wonders in the summer to keep humidity low, whereas in the winter humidity can be controlled with a dehumidifier. You may also want to consider installing a dehumidifier in your HVAC system.

A Danish study examined the impact of humidity control and ventilation on dust-mite concentrations in the home. At the beginning of the study, the dust-mite concentration was 110 mites per gram of mattress dust compared to 20 mites per gram after 4.7 months of routine ventilation. The authors concluded that "reduction of air humidity through an increased supply of fresh air may significantly diminish and, in some cases even eliminate, dust mites in homes."[6]

There are specific areas of your home that are prone to excess humidity. A damp basement is the perfect breeding ground for mold and mildew. Keep your basement clean and dry with a humidity level below 50 percent. You can place a dehumidifier in the basement or use a desiccant like Damp Check Dome Moisture Absorber that absorbs moisture. To determine whether your basement has a moisture problem, commercial kits can test for mold and mildew. If your home has a mold or mildew problem, there are many excellent anti-mold and -mildew products on the market like NAS-12, a remover, and No More Mildew, an inhibitor (both made by National Allergy Supply; 800-522-1448). Treat trouble areas with NAS-12 followed by a protective coating of No More Mildew. For do-it-yourself types, if you finish your basement, make sure the walls and floor are watertight and you have adequate ventilation and heating.

The bathroom is another humidity trouble spot, so it is especially important to thoroughly ventilate the bathroom daily, especially after a shower or bath. Also, regularly empty air conditioner, refrigerator, and dehumidifier water trays to keep your home's humidity levels low. This is especially important for air conditioners. While air-conditioning can significantly reduce mold and dust-mite concentrations in the home,[7] an improperly maintained air conditioner can act as a breeding ground for mold and cause serious trouble for sensitized asthmatics.

There are some parts of the country where the air is too dry. If you regularly use a humidifier, make sure to clean all its parts according to the manufacturer's recommendations and change the water daily. It is possible to catch some serious lung diseases from improperly maintained humidifiers. In fact, humidifiers have their own disease named for them—"humidifier fever."

CARPETING

Carpeting is off-limits for asthmatics, because of the amount of particulate matter that gets imbedded in the fibers. Especially dangerous is wet or damp carpeting, which acts as a breeding ground for mold. Dust mites also live in carpeting, especially in the bedroom. Multiple studies have documented that the higher the dust-mite concentration, the greater the risk of asthma. One Australian study found that the risk of asthma doubled for every doubling in the concentration of dust-mite allergen in sensitized individuals,[8] and another study found that the presence of dust mites increased the risk of asthma nearly eight times.[9]

Ideally, if you have asthma, your home should be carpet-free. Wood, tile, and stone flooring look wonderful, but can be expensive (there are laminated products that look like the real thing and are less pricey); linoleum is another option. If you already have wood, stone, tile, or linoleum floors, make sure you clean them with a damp mop regularly. You can also use an "electrostatic" dust cloth (such as Dust Grabber) that redistributes fewer allergens back into the air.

If you insist on carpeting, try area rugs and thoroughly clean them monthly. If you have wall-to-wall carpeting that you either will not or cannot remove, keep your carpet meticulously clean by vacuuming at least once a week and becoming a fanatic about source control.

Vacuuming a carpet is perhaps one of the most dangerous activities an asthmatic can perform. Every time you vacuum, you disperse into the air millions of bits of particulate pollution that can irritate your lungs. Complicating the problem is that standard vacuum-cleaner bags don't trap smaller particles (ten to twenty microns) and spew them back into the air. Even "water-based" vacuum cleaners only trap particles of ten microns or more. You might consider a high-efficiency vacuum cleaner with a HEPA filter.

One study examined sixty homes to measure how well high-efficiency vacuum cleaners removed cat, dog, and dust-mite allergens. While the authors found a "significant reduction" in cat dander and a modest reduction in dog dander, the vacuums did not significantly reduce dust-mite allergens. This study did, however, report that peak flow, FEV_1, and asthma symptoms improved after twelve months of using a high-efficiency vacuum cleaner. Interestingly, the study concluded that this improvement was "primarily achieved in those patients with cat sensitivity, but who did not possess a cat themselves."[10] What this means is that your neighbor's cat dander is floating through the air and landing in your house. Studies on school dust have found that it contains high levels of dog and cat allergens. Obviously a surprise to the superintendent who thought he was running a school and not a kennel—apparently, the animal dander was brought into the school on the children's clothing and shoes. So, if you think your home is safe from dog and cat dander, think again and consider getting a high-efficiency vacuum cleaner.

Now, what about those pesky dust mites? One study combined high-efficiency vacuum cleaning with mechanical ventilation and found a reduction in dust-mite allergens.[11] As with most asthma problems, source control is the best solution for dust mites. Keeping your home's humidity level under 50 percent will pull the dust-mite welcome mat away from the door. There are also carpet treatment products that reduce or kill dust mites: Allersearch X-Mite and Allersearch ADS neutralize dust mites, pet dander, and other allergens; DustMite and Flea Control, made by The Ecology Works, uses boron to kill dust mites and is registered with the EPA as safe for humans and pets.

Here's a recommendation I know you're going to like: There's no reason in the world for an asthmatic to vacuum a carpet. It is this doctor's order that when your carpet is being vacuumed, you leave the house. Make sure all windows are left open and your home is ventilated during and after vacuuming. The same advice applies to cleaning furniture, drapery, and carpeted and noncarpeted flooring, as well as to changing bed linens. Ventilating your home while cleaning helps disperse particulate pollution outside. Considering the value of your health, it may pay to hire someone to clean your home.

If you must vacuum, use a high-efficiency vacuum cleaner and make sure it is regularly serviced so that all its seals and connections remain airtight. An alternative to the traditional vacuum cleaner is a steam cleaner or vacuum cleaners that use steam to kill mites. Research comparing simple vacuuming to steam cleaning is scant, but one study from the National Institute of Environmental Health Sciences found that steam cleaning plus vacuuming and vacuuming alone resulted in a significant reduction in carpet dust-mite allergens.[12] Another study reported that carpet steam cleaning coupled with steam-heat cleaning of bedding and mattresses lowered dust-mite concentrations and resulted in a fourfold reduction of bronchial hyperreactivity in asthmatics.[13] If you use a steam cleaner, make sure to follow the manufacturer's instructions, as an overly wet carpet can promote mold and mildew, houseguests no asthmatic needs.

New carpeting is double-trouble for asthmatics. Not only will new carpet serve as a future allergen reservoir, but many asthmatics find the smell of new carpeting particularly bothersome. If you buy new carpeting, insist that the retailer unroll and ventilate the carpet prior to installation, and avoid using adhesives that emit noxious fumes. Also, bear in mind that carpeting directly applied to concrete often has moisture problems, especially basement carpeting. If you must carpet over concrete, insist on a moisture barrier. Try not to glue carpeting to the floor in case it becomes damaged and needs to be replaced or you decide to have it removed. The day the carpet is installed is a good day to be away. Finally, remember to completely ventilate your home for two to three days after carpet installation to help remove noxious fumes.

DRAPES, FURNITURE, AND HOUSEHOLD CLEANING

If you have textile window treatments, obey the same cleaning tips as for carpets, and treat your drapery with an anti-mildew and -mite agent. Consider using Allergex Dust Immobilizer, which, according to the manufacturer, prevents dust from being released into the air by trapping it in textiles. An alternative to textile window treatments are wood or plastic blinds and shades, which, in addition to being asthma-friendly, are stylish and practical.

Furniture fabrics can also trap allergens that aggravate asthma. Although it may be difficult to rid your home entirely of textiles—wood, metal, leather, and vinyl furniture are more asthma-friendly. How far you go in redecorating your home will depend on your symptoms, decorating tastes, and budget.

Cleaning and polishing wood and metal surfaces is another potential asthma hazard. Many household cleaners, polishers, and waxes contain organic chemicals that can trigger an asthma attack. The health risks of cleaning products continue even during storage, when dangerous fumes are released. According to the EPA, organic pollutant levels are two to five times higher inside the home than outside and people using these products expose themselves to high pollutant levels. In fact, elevated chemical concentrations linger in the air long after cleaning is completed.[14] Many of these chemicals, like benzene, have been found to cause cancer in humans.

With cleaning products, again source control is your best strategy, so you should store these products in an outdoor shed, airtight container, or your garage until needed. Conduct a complete search-and-destroy mission in your home and dispose of any outdated or unwanted cleaners and polishers. For information on household cleaning and polishing products, contact:

US Consumer Product Safety Commission (CPSC)
Washington, DC 20207-0001
Product Safety Hotline: 800-638-CPSC
Website: www.cpsc.gov

You can avoid chemical cleaners completely by using a simple damp cloth or an "electrostatic" dust collector (like the Dust Grabber) for dusting. There are even special dusting sprays like Allersearch AllerDust, designed to help the cloth attract dust and allergens. If you must use a chemical cleaner, carefully read the warnings and recommendations and thoroughly ventilate your house during and after use. When practical, clean household items outdoors—easy for a toaster oven, a bit more challenging for an armoire.

BEDROOM

We think of the bedroom as a refuge, but for some asthmatics the bedroom is the most dangerous room in the house. It contains that dreaded piece of furniture that strikes fear in the lungs of asthmatics—the bed. You spend about a third of your life in bed and, while you sleep, you are shedding skin. Shed skin serves as dust-mite food. As we have seen, asthmatics have a major problem with dust mites. Unfortunately, dust mites are a fact of life and have nothing to do with how clean you keep your home. As long as there's skin, there will be dust mites. Not only do we sleep in dust-mite heaven, every time you or your loved one makes the slightest movement, your mattress, box springs, pillows, sheets, and blankets get ruffled and release dust-mite allergens into the air.

What can you do? Because a concrete bed probably isn't appealing to you, I suggest covering your pillows, mattress, comforters, and box springs in special fabrics called "encasements," which are designed to minimize the amount of dust-mite allergens released into the air. Even "hypoallergenic" bedding needs to be encased as it is not dust mite-proof. Encasements used to be made of plastics that were noisy and uncomfortable, but now there are quality cotton and polyester encasements that are quiet and soft.

One study examined twenty-four children with asthma who encased their mattresses, blankets, and pillows and treated their bedroom carpets with tannic acid, which kills dust mites. After eight months, there was a significant reduction in bronchial hyperreactivity.[15] Another group of researchers studied twenty asthmatics who encased their pillows, mattresses, and box springs, while simultaneously washing blankets, mattress pads, and curtains every two weeks. Their bedrooms were kept as clean and dust-free as possible and, after one month, there was a significant difference in asthma symptoms. Those with dust-free bedrooms had fewer days on which they wheezed, took medication, or had an abnormal peak expiratory flow rate. Specifically, wheezing was recorded on only 2 percent of the days, compared to 27 percent in the control group; days on which medication was required dropped from 30 percent to 2 percent; and low peak flow occurred on 1 percent of days, versus 28 percent in the control group. The dust-free group also had a fourfold increase in their ability to tolerate histamine. The authors concluded that "a dust-free bedroom diminishes bronchial irritability and is a practical and effective method for decreasing asthma in children with house dust or house dust mite allergy."[16]

Maintaining a dust-free bedroom may also help prevent asthma in infants. One study examined the effect of having fifty-eight breast-feeding mothers and their infants abstain from eating allergenic foods (milk, eggs, fish, and nuts), while treating the child's bedroom with a mite-killing powder every three months until the child's first birthday. A control group of sixty-two mother-infant pairs had no dietary restrictions or bedroom treatments. After twelve months, allergic disease was diagnosed in 40 percent of the control group compared to 13 percent of the treatment group.[17]

By the way, breast-feeding mothers should consider avoiding common allergenic foods for the first twelve months of their infant's life while keeping their child's solid diet free of dairy products, eggs, fish, nuts, oranges, wheat, and unhydrolyzed soya for the first nine months. One study reported that these interventions helped protect infants from asthma.[18]

So, get rid of dust mites and you'll probably feel better. If you can't find encasements locally, check the Allergy Buyers Club, a supplier of asthma- and allergy-friendly products such as bedding, laundry detergents, air filters, pet products, home-cleaning products, vacuum cleaners, and anti-mite and -allergen supplies. The Allergy Buyers Club also has an informative website. You can contact them at:

Allergy Buyers Club
161 North Street
Newtonville, MA 02460
Phone: 888-236-7231 • Fax: 617-332-0292
Website: www.AllergyBuyersClub.com

Another supplier of allergy and asthma products is the Allergy Supply Company:

Allergy Supply Company
11994 Star Court
Herndon, VA 20171
Phone: 800-323-6744 • Fax: 703-391-2014
Website: www.allergysupply.com

One more recommended source of asthma-related products is Allergy One:

Allergy One
PO Box 28302
Fresno, CA 93729-8302
Phone: 559-432-1900 • Fax: 559-432-1910
Website: www.allergyone.com

The dust mites that inhabit your mattress also live on your sheets and blankets. To make the life of a dust mite especially miserable, wash your sheets, blankets, pillow covers, comforters, and mattress pads every ten to fourteen days in hot (130°F) water. Consider using Allersearch Allergen Wash or De-Mite laundry additive, which can be added to your wash to kill dust mites and remove allergens. You may also want to consider buying asthma-friendly fleece blankets made of Vellux. In case you don't believe dust mites are sharing your home, there is an inexpensive test called Aclotest, made by Allergy Laboratories of Ohio Inc., which can measure your dust-mite population.

One additional asthma problem may be hanging in your bedroom closet. Dry cleaners often use perchloroethylene, an organic chemical that may cause cancer. If your clothes have a strong chemical odor after dry cleaning, return them to your cleaner for proper care. If your asthma is triggered by the smell of dry-cleaned clothing, have your clothes washed rather than dry-cleaned.

BATHROOM

The bathroom can be a scary place if smells exacerbate your asthma. Humans have an overwhelming need to mask their natural odors, something clearly reflected in the wide variety of personal grooming products. Since most of these products are scented and represent potential asthma triggers, I suggest temporarily placing all toiletries in an outside storage shed or the garage. This will give your lungs a break and you can see if your breathing gets better. Don't worry, you'll be able to present yourself in public one day! We will gradually reintroduce this stuff back into your life to discover which products cause your asthma to flare up.

What about the necessities? Toilet paper is a necessity, so use scentless toilet tissue. Also available are scentless soaps, free of dyes, formaldehyde, lanolin, parabens, and perfumes, all of which can cause trouble in susceptible asthmatics. There are even asthma-friendly hair-care products, such as Free & Clear shampoo and conditioner. Other than these necessities, try to exile your toiletry collection from your home on the weekends and see how your lungs react. Ideally, you should go one month without toiletries to give your lungs time to recover. After four weeks, introduce one personal grooming product back into your life every three days. Take two good whiffs of each product prior to bringing it back home; if your asthma flares up, then perhaps it's time to change or eliminate that product.

Most people want to resume using toothpaste and underarm deodorant as soon as possible. Toothpaste usually doesn't cause trouble, although some asthmatics are sensitive to the mint odor. There are retailers who offer scentless, nontoxic personal care products (toothpaste, shampoo, deodorant, and hair conditioner) for people with asthma, allergies, and chemical sensitivities. (For more information on these products, visit the Health Cybernetics website: www.healthcybernetics.com/pure.htm.)

There are several odorless skin moisturizers, such as Vanicream (made by Pharmaceutical Specialists, Inc.). Also available are sunscreens that don't contain benzophenone, dyes, formaldehyde, lanolin, PABA, perfumes, and preservatives. Be wary of lotions that are "fragrance-free"—this means there is no heavy perfume, but it does not mean the product is odorless or entirely free of additives that may cause asthma trouble. For people with sensitivities, the more toiletries you add to your life, the more likely you are to have a reaction. You can learn which grooming products you can and cannot tolerate by keeping a careful diary of what you use and how you react.

Finally, if you like to leave the toothpaste cap off, you should be aware that roaches adore toothpaste, even sniffing your toothbrush for residue. To keep roaches out of your bathroom, cap the toothpaste after every use and seal your toothbrush in a roach-proof container.

LAUNDRY ROOM

The laundry room contains many potential asthma triggers: fabric softeners, scented laundry detergents, and dust and lint that don't quite make it out through the dryer vent. Like the rest of your home, keep the laundry room meticulously clean and dust-free. Always shut the laundry room door when washing or drying clothes and, if there is a door or window between the laundry room and the garage or outside, keep it open to allow dust and fumes to escape. Until you figure out exactly what triggers your asthma, I recommend using unscented detergents and fabric softeners.

KITCHEN

The kitchen is a hot asthma trouble spot. In the kitchen, asthmatics have to contend with cooking smells and products of combustion. Although cooking with gas is relatively clean, natural gas combustion still delivers an oxidative load to the lungs. If you cook with gas, be sure the flame is blue not yellow—a yellow flame signals inefficient burning and increased pollution. If you're planning to buy a gas stove, insist on "pilotless ignition" so you don't have a pilot light burning continuously.

Ventilation is critical in the kitchen. For both electric and gas stoves, make sure you have a properly working exhaust fan and hood that vents smoke and cooking fumes and sends them outside. If you like to cook and spend a lot of time in the kitchen, consider installing a high-efficiency, multispeed exhaust system over the stove. In addition to using an exhaust fan, keep your kitchen windows open and doors closed when cooking. If you have the luxury of designing a new home or redesigning your kitchen, install kitchen doors to prevent cooking fumes from spilling into the rest of your home. Cooking outdoors is the ultimate solution, but remember to keep your home's windows closed so fumes don't drift in.

By paying careful attention to your asthma symptoms and how they relate to cooking smells, you can quickly learn which odors are safe and which are not. Of course, eating at a nice restaurant is a great way to avoid cooking smells; however, this can get pricey. Most asthmatics do fine in a well-ventilated kitchen.

Besides being a haven for odors, the kitchen is also a favorite hangout for cockroaches. People living in large cities generally have the most roach problems. From personal experience, I know that many city folk, no matter how roach-proof their own kitchen, cannot control "the cockroach breeder king" who happens to live next door. What follows is some helpful advice on how to keep that brood from invading your home.

New York City and Chicago didn't get to lead the nation in asthma because of bad air alone: they have more cockroaches than you can count. It's no secret that roach feces and body parts are major contributors to asthma in many inner-city communities. A 1997 report from the National Cooperative Inner-City Asthma Study found that the degree of cockroach exposure was related to the risk of hospitalization for asthma in children.[19] Cockroaches and their droppings are classic asthma triggers. You can avoid the ubiquitous roach by keeping your kitchen spotless and roach-proofing your home. This means no open food products in your cabinets or refrigerator. Place anything that might tempt the inquisitive roach—from an open box of cereal to fresh cheese to spices—in tightly sealed plastic or glass containers.

You can also control the roach population by eating all your meals in the kitchen or dining room, thereby preventing roach breeding in other parts of the house. Take the trash out nightly and never leave dirty dishes in the sink. Every night, make sure the sink is absolutely spotless and the dishwasher door is closed and locked. Clean appliances that may harbor food crumbs, such as the oven, microwave, toaster, stovetop, and blender, after each use.

This aggressive form of source control is the most effective way to keep roaches out of your home. Depending on where you live and who your neighbors are, you may not be able to completely eliminate roaches, but these simple measures will help make your home an inhospitable place for roaches.

LIVING ROOM

Like the bedroom, the living room is a major allergen reservoir, with upholstered furniture and carpeting acting as dust and allergen magnets. See the previous sections on carpeting and furniture for helpful cleaning tips.

The living room may also have a fireplace, which produces products of combustion, such as carbon monoxide, nitrogen dioxide, and gobs of particulate matter. If you have a fireplace or wood stove, make certain there is adequate ventilation and that the units are maintained regularly. Use only aged, cured wood and never burn pressure-treated wood. If you have a gas fireplace, you still have to open the flue during use. Besides being fire hazards, dirty flues and chimneys are a major source of gaseous and particulate air pollution. Even worse, a poorly maintained flue or chimney can cause deadly levels of carbon monoxide to accumulate in your home. Make sure your chimney and flue are cleaned regularly and follow all maintenance instructions.

The same advice applies to kerosene and other types of space heaters. When using a space heater, always follow the manufacturer's directions, use only the recommended fuel, and keep the room's door slightly ajar and windows cracked open to insure adequate ventilation.

DINING ROOM

The dining room is often a victim of circumstance, given its proximity to the kitchen with its high concentration of cooking odors and combustion products. Ventilating your kitchen goes a long way toward keeping your dining room asthma-friendly. With the exception of carpeting and upholstered furniture, there is little in most dining rooms that can trigger an asthma attack. Beware, however, of floral or fragrant table arrangements that may cause trouble, especially during holidays.

YOUR CHILD'S ROOM

I don't need to tell you that neatness and childhood often don't mix. However, if you or your child has asthma, it is important that your child's room stays as clean as the rest of the house. Even if your children don't have asthma, you should still encase and regularly wash their bedding to control dust mites. Every now and then, check under your child's bed for dust balls, and do a quick search for unauthorized pets. Be aware that your older children's scented grooming products may also aggravate your asthma.

STUDY OR DEN

In addition to heeding the warnings about carpeting and upholstered furniture, be aware that the den is often the site of potentially toxic hobby supplies. Airplane glue, solvents, paints, and plastics can trigger an asthma attack. Carefully consider what you do in the den with special attention to your hobbies. If you discover that you own potentially noxious hobby or craft supplies, treat these products just like cleaning agents: immediately exile them outdoors, and gradually reintroduce them to your home, meticulously recording associated symptoms.

GARAGE

Most garages are packed with potentially toxic substances, such as pesticides, fertilizers, cleaning supplies, oil and gasoline, paint cans, and cat-litter boxes. Ideally, this toxic material is best stored in a ventilated outdoor storage shed, with the garage being the storage site of last resort. Look for chemicals, cleaners, and gardening supplies you no longer use and get rid of them. (Check with your local health department for the proper disposal of these items.)

Also, don't let your car idle in the garage, as exhaust fumes can find their way into your home. Finally, make sure your car's ventilation ducts and air conditioner are regularly maintained with frequent filter replacement, since asthma may be exacerbated by a contaminated air-conditioning system.

ATTIC, BASEMENT, OR CRAWLSPACE

The attic, basement, and crawlspaces are the places where we store—and forget about—all sorts of items, such as chemicals, cans of paint, and old clothing. Mothballs and moth repellent are additional potent triggers that can aggravate asthma. Keep the humidity of these spaces under 50 percent, periodically check for mold and mildew, and try to keep dust to a minimum. While examining your attic, you may be surprised to learn that birds and other critters have taken up residence under your roof. While small mammals need a place to live, the home of an asthmatic should not be one of them. Birds and rodents bring in or "drop" feces, feathers, and dirt that may irritate your lungs. So, give your furry, feathered friends a gentle "heave-ho" back to nature where they belong.

PLANTS AND GARDENS

If you're a gardener, consider wearing a mask while doing yard work so you don't inhale soil and plant allergens. Overgrown plants and shrubs are potential asthma offenders that should be kept under control. If you're allergic to grass, it pays to have someone else mow your lawn. Houseplants are another source of asthma trouble. Contrary to popular belief, houseplants do not remove indoor air pollution. The pollen they release and the mold that can grow in their damp soil may actually aggravate your asthma.

PETS

Pets are leading contributors to asthma-related illness. Nobody said this was going to be easy, but before you jump to any conclusions, I am not going to insist that you give up your pet. Chances are you love your pet as much as you love your family. I do suggest, however, that you take a critical look at the potential health consequences of owning a pet. Before you can make a decision, we must first determine if you're allergic to your pet or a pet-related product. As I shared with you in the Introduction, my asthma began with a rabbit. In reality, the rabbit didn't aggravate my asthma at all—the cedar chips in the rabbit's litter box did. This is why discovering what triggers your asthma is so critical. Some pet owners may find that their pet has nothing to do with their symptoms; rather, their lungs react to a pet-related product. Other asthmatics may unfortunately discover that they would not have asthma were it not for their pet.

For most asthmatics, when it comes to pets, the major offender is either a dog or cat. While both can get an asthmatic into trouble, cats pose the most danger because feline dander is more allergenic. Cat dander is also smaller, therefore likely to stay airborne longer. Skin testing can help determine if you're allergic to your pet, especially if you have a strong reaction. Skin testing, however, is not always accurate.

You may need a trial separation from your pet. Though it may be emotionally difficult, leave your pet with a friend or pet-care professional for one month and completely remove all pet-related products from your home. You'll also need to eliminate residual dander by thoroughly cleaning your home and washing all clothes, linens, and carpeting. It is also vital that during this separation you follow the advice detailed later in this chapter regarding the total removal of asthma triggers from your home. A meticulously planned removal of all allergens, followed by a top to bottom cleaning of your home, has a greater chance of success than removing items one by one.

This is when keeping an asthma diary becomes critically important, so you can determine if your symptoms abate while your pet is away. If after four weeks your symptoms don't improve, chances are Fido isn't to blame. Conversely, if your asthma miraculously disappears while your pet is away, you will have a difficult decision to make. If you find that your pet is causing your asthma, you will have to decide what is more important—protecting your health or having a pet. For the sake of your own well-being, you may need to find your pet another loving home. On an intellectual level you understand this, but on an emotional level it's a different story.

If the thought of giving up a pet is unthinkable, there are several steps you can take to protect yourself. First, seriously consider keeping your pet and all pet-related products outdoors. If you cannot or will not keep your pet outside, then at least restrict your pet's access to as few rooms as possible. Designate one room as a "pet room," making sure this space is adequately ventilated, has an air cleaner or purifier, and is damp-mopped weekly, at a minimum. Make sure your home has several HEPA air cleaners, as these high-efficiency filters can significantly reduce animal dander. Insure that whatever your pet sleeps on and plays with is laundered or cleaned weekly. Keep your pet out of the bedroom and never let a pet sleep with you. As you already know, the bedroom is a dangerous place for asthmatics and your pet only makes the situation worse. Be sure to wash your pet twice weekly, since a clean pet leaves behind less dander; one study found that airborne dog allergens were reduced 84 percent by washing the dog twice weekly.[20] There are products, such as PetWize Cat and Dog Allergen Control and skin moisturizers, that can be applied to your pet's fur to reduce dander.

Even though there are alternatives to pet problems, my professional advice is that it would be wise to put your pet elsewhere. While there are some asthmatics who are sensitive to only a specific allergen, most asthmatics are sensitive to multiple allergens and it is difficult to discover every asthma trigger. Keeping a diary remains critical and will hopefully help you identify and remove many triggers. There are, however, subtle triggers that we may not be aware of but can nonetheless cause trouble. This is why I strongly advocate removing pets from your home. Even if your symptoms did not improve during your pet's trial separation, you may still be allergic to animal dander. One study examined two groups of asthmatics: one with dogs or cats, the other without. According to the study, more people with pets had symptoms (abnormal peak flow, higher eosinophil counts, and greater bronchial hyperresponsiveness) and used steroids than subjects without pets.[21] While a pet may not be entirely responsible for your symptoms, there's a good chance your pet is contributing to your asthma.

Think hard and make a basic life decision: Do I risk my health for a pet? I cannot make the decision for you; this tough choice is up to you.

YOUR HOME'S HIDDEN DANGER: FORMALDEHYDE

Found in the resin that holds particleboard together, formaldehyde is a known asthma trigger that may cause cancer. Particleboard is a building material made from wood chips that are pressed and glued together with resin. Formaldehyde enters the environment and your lungs as it is released from the resin. Particleboard is commonly used in furniture, cabinetry, and new-home construction. While the quantity of formaldehyde emitted by a product usually decreases with time, for asthmatics it is best to buy furniture and cabinets made from non-pressed wood or "exterior grade" building materials that emit less formaldehyde. If you own furniture made of particleboard, you can apply a coat of polyurethane to help reduce formaldehyde emissions. Because fresh polyurethane fumes can trigger an asthma attack, apply polyurethane outside and allow it to dry completely before returning the product to your home. If you suspect your home has a formaldehyde problem, keep your house cool and dry to reduce the emission rate, since formaldehyde emission is accelerated by heat and humidity.

If you're building or remodeling a home, remember that plywood, particleboard, and insulation may contain formaldehyde. To reduce formaldehyde emissions, talk to your builder about solid wood construction or formaldehyde "poor" building materials, like exterior-grade pressed wood. Also, if you live in a new or recently renovated home, pay special attention to routine ventilation for the first two to three years. If you're building a new home, consider installing a mechanical ventilation system or an air-to-air heat exchanger. Besides formaldehyde-containing building materials, home renovations can be particularly hazardous to asthmatics because of the dust and fumes generated by remodeling. If practical, try to stay away from home during active construction and make sure your house remains ventilated and dust-free. If you want to learn more about formaldehyde or check on the safety of a particular product, call the EPA Toxic Substances Control Act Line at 202-554-1404.

YOUR WORKPLACE

While the primary focus of this chapter is the home, your workplace may also be aggravating your symptoms. Besides respiratory symptoms, office buildings can cause nausea, fatigue, sneezing, and a number of other symptoms generally referred to as "building-related illnesses" or "sick building syndrome." Modern office buildings that boast controlled envi-

A Step-by-Step Action Plan for Creating an Asthma-Safe Environment

The purpose of this chapter is to help you create an asthma-safe environment by removing those substances that are notorious for triggering and perpetuating asthma. While following these recommendations will not guarantee an asthma-free life, many of you will experience a significant improvement in your symptoms. Let's now use this information to formulate an action plan for creating an asthma-friendly home.

First, search your entire home, room by room, and make a list of all potential asthma triggers, such as cleaning agents, chemicals, and personal-care products. Discard immediately those items that are outdated or no longer used. Once you have a list, set a date one month later on which you will rid your home of as many asthma triggers as possible. On that day, have your entire home cleaned, preferably by a professional cleaning company. Pay special attention to textile products, which are notorious allergen reservoirs. Remember, even if your pet is on a trial separation, the dander is still hiding in your carpet, furniture, and drapes. Have all drapery, comforters, rugs, linens, and window treatments professionally laundered. If you have a roach problem, carefully examine your kitchen and identify trouble spots; you may need to bring in an exterminator.

Inform your family of your cleaning plans—asthma is not just your problem, it's everyone's problem. You'll need your family's support and cooperation, especially after they learn you intend to eliminate personal-grooming products for a month. Your family should understand that, for a month after the house is cleaned and fumigated, they are not to bring any new nonfood items into the home without your permission. As you can imagine, this takes planning, so let's develop a checklist.

Two to Three Weeks Before Cleaning Day

You need to take several steps prior to cleaning day:

1. Make a list of all potential asthma triggers in your home, including:
    - Auto-care products
    - Chemicals
    - Cleaning products
        - Glass cleaner
        - Furniture polish/cleaner

  - Laundry detergent
  - Soaps and shampoos
- Garden supplies
- Personal care and grooming items
- Pets and pet-related products

2. You need to purchase the following:
   - Anti-mite carpet and laundry additives
   - Encasements for your mattress, box springs, pillows, and comforters
   - Filters for the furnace, air conditioner, and air cleaners
   - Food-storage containers to eliminate roach problems
   - Scent-free laundry detergent, soap, and shampoo
   - Outdoor storage shed
3. Make some phone calls:
   - Arrange pet care
   - Hire a professional cleaning company (Explain what you're doing. Tell them you need to have the following cleaned: all carpeting, curtains and drapery, furniture, walls, ceilings, and floors. They should also pay special attention to signs of mold and mildew.)

On Cleaning Day

Banish all potential asthma triggers to an outdoor storage shed (or the garage), send your pet to off-site care, and have your home completely cleaned. Launder all clothing and linens with scent-free detergent using hot water and anti-mite treatment; dry-clean those items you cannot launder. Have all your comforters and blankets professionally cleaned. Stay away from home while the cleaning company is working, since intense cleaning can release tremendous amounts of particulate and odorous pollutants. Make sure all carpets are thoroughly cleaned and treated with an anti-mite agent. Once your home is cleaned, immediately remove and discard all air filters and open every window and vent for one full day. If possible, stay in a hotel that night. After you ventilate your home, install new air filters and encase your mattress, box springs, pillows, and comforters. Finally, establish a ban on bringing new potential asthma triggers into your home.

One Month after Cleaning Day

By this time, you should be feeling better and your family would no doubt like to have their stuff back. Gradually reintroduce potential asthma triggers back into your home, while paying close attention to how your asthma reacts. I suggest you reintroduce a new item every three to four days. If your asthma acts up two hours after bringing a particular product into the house, you know it is part of the problem. Since most asthmatics are sensitive to multiple agents, don't be surprised if you find several items that need to be permanently exiled. Prior to bringing a potential trigger inside your house, take two good whiffs of that item. If your lungs react, you know that product will have to be eliminated.

Consider permanently keeping all cleaning agents, auto-care products, and chemicals in a separate outdoor storage area. Even if you don't react to these products, it does not mean their fumes do not impact your asthma. Furthermore, the fumes generated by these products represent a constant stress on your lungs and can have a negative effect on other organs. So, with the exception of items you safely use every day, anything that has the potential to release gaseous pollution is probably best kept outside your home.

If this cleaning process does not help you discover what is triggering your asthma, consider hiring a company that specializes in indoor air-quality evaluations. Check the Yellow Pages under the heading "Air Quality—Indoor." While there will always be the rare idiopathic asthmatic, I believe most of you will breathe easier after cleaning and ridding your home of potential asthma triggers.

ronments and airtight windows can unwittingly permit potentially dangerous indoor air pollution levels to develop. According to the World Health Organization, up to 30 percent of new or remodeled commercial buildings may have unusually high rates of health complaints related to indoor air quality.[22]

Take a moment to reflect: When is your asthma worse, at home or at work? If you answered "at work," you may have occupational asthma. The air at work may contain a variety of particulate and chemical pollutants usually not found in private homes and apartments. The list of substances that may cause occupational asthma is extensive, so if your asthma is worse at work, you'll need to put on your detective cap and hunt for suspects.

One potentially quick solution for work-related asthma is to determine if your building has a ventilation system that exchanges outside air for inside air. If so, check your office to see if the input/output vents are blocked or not working. The simple act of insuring adequate office ventilation can solve many breathing problems. If you discover the source of your asthma trouble, notify management of your findings in the most politically sensitive way possible; you may be surprised at how cooperative they are. The EPA publishes an excellent guide to office air quality entitled *An Office Building Occupant's Guide to Indoor Air Quality* EPA-402-K-97-003 (Washington, DC: US EPA, October 1997), which you can find on the Internet (www.epa.gov/iaq/pubs/occupgd.html) or by calling 800-438-4318.

Information regarding evaluation and/or inspection of your office can be obtained through the National Institute for Occupational Safety and Health (NIOSH) by calling 800-356-4674 or by writing or calling:

Occupational Safety and Health Administration (OSHA)
Office of Information and Consumer Affairs
200 Constitution Avenue, NW, Room N-3647
Washington, DC 20210
Phone: 800-321-OSHA
Website: www.osha.gov

While most employers will cooperate to correct work-related air-quality problems, there may be circumstances in which notifying a federal or state agency is appropriate. This is especially true when there are multiple complaints of work-related illness that remain unexplained or when an employer refuses to correct an obviously hazardous situation.

chapter 7

Vitamin, Mineral, and Dietary Supplements

When I started writing about integrative medicine several years ago, I was skeptical about vitamins, minerals, and herbs, or any therapy that didn't involve high technology or at least a powerful pharmaceutical. As I researched various alternative therapies, it dawned on me that many of them really worked. I was pleasantly surprised to learn that the people who researched alternative therapies came from backgrounds similar to my own and experienced the same difficulties every scientist faces when seeking the truth. It has been a profound learning experience that has forever changed the way I look at health and medicine. So, before we delve into the subject of supplements for asthma, let us briefly examine the challenges and problems that scientists face when conducting research.

THE CHALLENGES OF NUTRITIONAL RESEARCH

Nutrient deficiencies usually occur in one of three ways: inadequate intake, improper absorption, or increased demand. In asthmatics, it appears that persistent internal and external oxidative stress and decreased dietary intake play the most important roles in vitamin and mineral deficiencies. Knowing this, investigators have conducted research into vitamin and mineral supplements to determine if replacing a deficient agent can improve or eliminate asthma. One of the problems with supplement research is that if an individual is deficient in substance A, chances are they are also deficient in substances X, Y, and Z. In other words, vitamin and mineral deficiencies do not occur in a vacuum; the dietary or medical derangements that created the original deficiency usually cause other deficiencies. This is why it is difficult to study one particular deficiency without taking into consideration others.

Further complicating the picture, proper lung function rests not on a single nutrient but on an entire symphony of vitamins and minerals that are responsible for overall health. This is why it is difficult to test the impact on asthma of supplementation with a particular vitamin or mineral. For instance, researchers attempting to determine the effect of vitamin C on asthma may take a group of asthmatics deficient in vitamin C and correct their deficiency through supplementation. The problem is that while the vitamin C deficiency may be corrected, there are probably additional nutrient deficiencies contributing to the asthma. Despite these limitations, research has demonstrated that specific nutrient supplements do help asthmatics.

As you read this chapter, you will notice that most researchers report that a particular supplement benefited some but not all study participants. This is a common finding because the medical condition we call "asthma" is the shared endpoint of multiple abnormal biological pathways. Each asthmatic has a unique set of genetic, environmental, and psychological influences, which is why we have multiple types of asthma that often respond to different treatments. Multiple asthmatic pathways present a special challenge to researchers who are still in the process of understanding how they work and interact. Asthma clearly results from a complex interplay between genes and environment causing us to see a particular supplement work for some but not all asthmatics. As our knowledge grows, we are beginning to understand that, while many roads lead to asthma, they tend to end at the same place, and we are finding that the most successful therapies are those that target these common pathways, such as leukotriene synthesis.

Nutrient researchers also have to contend with different diets among study subjects. The ideal supplement study would examine two groups of people with identical medical conditions, nutrient deficiencies, and diets while comparing the effect of supplementation versus no supplementation. Though we can find people with similar medical conditions, it's difficult to control and monitor individual diets. With animal studies, you can totally control an animal's diet and the integrity of the study data. The tough part about human-diet studies is that people cheat. While scientists have mathematical models that correct data for different diets, dietary aberrations will always remain a potential source of error.

EVIDENCE-BASED MEDICINE

Doctors use many therapies because they work, not because there are multiple scientific studies documenting that a particular treatment is superior to another. We are all, in part, a product of our history, and modern medicine is no exception. Mercifully, physicians also learn from their mistakes and when a treatment does more harm than good, it is quickly abandoned.

Over the past decade, physicians have begun to realize that it's not good enough to choose a therapy just because it's the one they have always used to treat a given condition. Such concern has resulted in a revolution called "evidence-based medicine" (EBM), a relatively new and exciting chapter in medical history. EBM demands that therapies make scientific sense and are rigorously tested to see if they actually offer benefit.

One of the fundamental tenets of EBM is that the best way to test whether a treatment works is to take a group of people with medical condition X and randomly divide them into treatment group A and placebo group B, with neither doctor nor patient knowing who is in each group, and then see how they do. This basic technique is used in what is called a double-blind, randomized, placebo-controlled trial (RCT), the preferred evidence-based research design. With RCTs, the larger the population, the more you can generalize the results. This is not to say that small study groups make for a bad trial; it only means that, in general, the more participants the better.

There is one more study design you should know about: the meta-analysis. Meta-analysis is considered one of the most powerful EBM tools. While RCTs examine individual groups of patients, meta-analysis examines the validity of multiple RCTs. Put another way, meta-analysis critically analyzes a group of RCTs, examining them for the quality of their design, and then offers a summary of their pooled conclusions.

OTHER RESEARCH CONSIDERATIONS

Most of the studies mentioned in this book are human trials. Animal studies are important, especially for trials that enter uncharted, potentially dangerous waters; but human studies remain the gold standard, since there are important differences between animals and humans that may influence results.

With respect to asthma research, results are usually reported as objective or subjective findings. Objective findings are variables that can be measured using standardized instruments and are therefore reproducible. Typical objective findings in asthma research include peak flow, FEV, and FEV_1. Subjective findings are "quality of life" scores, calculated from a standardized survey. While peak flow, FEV, and FEV_1 can be influenced by patient effort, these variables are generally considered more indicative of treatment success or failure than subjective findings.

Another variable commonly reported by asthma researchers, which shares elements of both subjective and objective findings, is medication use. While we can objectively measure how much medicine an asthmatic is using, a patient's decision to increase or decrease medication usually depends on subjective feelings of how their asthma is doing rather than on actual lung function.

The physician in me likes objective findings, since these are quantitative variables that indicate how a treatment is working. As an asthmatic, all I care about is how well I feel. In the end, subjective and objective findings are equally important. While it is vital to measure objective improvement in lung function, the most important therapy variable for the asthmatic is "Do I feel better?"

Finally, in Chapter 4, we discussed the stages of scientific research—from initial hypothesis to intense research, publication, and controversy to final acceptance, rejection, or revision. While the concept of diet affecting health and asthma is generally accepted, we remain in the research-publication-controversy stage when it comes to individual supplements for asthma. Some supplements, like vitamin C, have accumulated a substantial body of literature supporting their use. For other supplements, research is intense and findings are hotly debated.

VITAMIN AND MINERAL SUPPLEMENTATION 101

As with any emerging field of medicine, controversy exists over the true impact supplements can have on asthma. Nevertheless, there is a substantial body of literature indicating that vitamin and mineral supplementation helps many asthmatics. While there is no substitute for a healthy diet coupled with adequate sleep and exercise, nutrient supplements have become a necessity in our increasingly toxic world. Our toxic environment routinely delivers an excessive oxidant load that frequently overwhelms the body's antioxidant defenses. Furthermore, research has shown that asthmatics are often antioxidant deficient. Given these considerations, every asthmatic should routinely supplement their diet with antioxidants.

My personal favorites are vitamin C and coenzyme Q_{10}, which I take every morning with a multivitamin. Ask a knowledgeable healthcare professional to help you choose the antioxidants that are right for your individual needs. For instance, if your family has a history of heart disease and high cholesterol, vitamin C would be an excellent choice because it is the lung's primary antioxidant and studies have shown that it reduces cholesterol. If you're worried about prostate cancer, consider taking selenium, a powerful antioxidant shown to help asthmatics and reduce the risk of prostate cancer.

I recommend supplementing your diet with two antioxidants that will help your asthma and also protect you against the diseases for which you're personally at risk. Chances are your breathing will improve after one to two months of taking these antioxidants. After two months, if your breathing does not improve, continue taking your standard antioxidant supplements while experimenting with additional vitamins or minerals for asthma relief. Give each supplement a four-week trial, recording symptoms in your asthma diary. I also suggest you get tested for vitamin and mineral deficiencies and, with the aid of a healthcare professional, correct any deficiency found.

Remember that nutritional supplements are only a small part of the asthma picture. The purpose of this book is to eliminate or markedly improve your asthma. The foundation of good health and proper lung function rests not with supplements alone; rather, a healthy life demands a clean environment, good nutrition, regular exercise, and adequate sleep. Supplements can certainly help the asthmatic, but they are only one piece of a complex puzzle we call health.

Vitamin A (retinol)

You'll realize the benefits of vitamin A if you're reading this book at night, since without retinol you would not be able to see this page. Vitamin A helps us see in dim light, and a deficiency can result in night blindness. Vitamin A also keeps epithelial cells, which line the airways and act as a vital line of defense against bacteria and viruses, intact. Vitamin A can stimulate immune function as well, helping to fight infections. Vitamin A helps cells grow normally, which becomes important in cancer protection since a fundamental cancer mechanism is deranged cell growth. Despite being a relatively weak antioxidant, vitamin A is used to treat several conditions, including night blindness, measles, acne, and celiac disease.

Research shows that vitamin A deficiency negatively impacts the lungs by playing a role in the shift from Th1 to Th2 T-cells. This shift results in increased levels of leukotrienes and prostaglandin E_2, major chemical mediators of the asthma cascade. Particularly striking is that when the lungs of retinol-deficient animals are examined, they exhibit many of the pathologic changes seen in cigarette smokers. In a 2002 study at the University of Iowa, researchers found that the lungs of vitamin-A-deficient rats were more responsive to methacholine.[1] Other studies have demonstrated that low blood levels of vitamin A carry an increased risk of airway obstruction in humans.[2] The fact that smokers who drink milk have a lower risk of bronchitis has led some researchers to suspect that high vitamin A intake may protect the lungs.[3]

This association between vitamin A deficiency and airway disease was supported by researchers at Johns Hopkins University. They examined data from over 3,800 individuals who participated in the First National Health and Nutrition Examination Survey (NHANES I) and concluded that a diet poor in vitamin A increases the risk of airway obstruction.[4] Further strengthening this relationship is a British study demonstrating that "brittle" asthmatics have low dietary vitamin A, with an average intake of 522.5 micrograms per day compared to 806.5 mcg/day in healthy adults.[5] Why retinol deficiency is a risk factor for asthma remains the subject of intense investigation; however, a possible explanation may be that vitamin A inhibits eosinophils and basophils, which play a role in histamine release.[6]

Dietary sources: Vitamin A is found in fruits, meat, liver, poultry, vegetables, dairy products, and cod liver oil. Beta-carotene, a powerful antioxidant carotenoid found in vegetables and fruits, can be converted to vitamin A in the body.

Dosage: Most authorities typically recommend 10,000–25,000 IU of vitamin A daily for long-term supplementation. Since only a small percentage of beta-carotene is converted to vitamin A, beta-carotene supplements should not result in retinol toxicity. Vitamin A is best absorbed when taken with food.

Side effects: Toxicity is usually only seen in daily doses over 25,000 IU. Side effects include abdominal pain, bone loss, dry skin, fatigue, gingivitis, inflammation of the lips and tongue, hair loss, headaches, high cholesterol, itching, joint pain, liver injury, loss of appetite, nausea, night sweats, and vomiting.

Precautions during pregnancy: If you're pregnant or lactating, speak to your doctor before taking a vitamin A supplement.

Drug interactions: Interactions with atorvastatin, colestipol, corticosteroids, cyclophosphamide, fluvastatin, isotretinoin, lovastatin, medroxyprogesterone, methyltestosterone, mineral oil, minocycline, neomycin, pravastatin, simvastatin, thioridazine, and tretinoin have been reported. Interactions have also been found with chemotherapy drugs, oral contraceptives, bile-acid binding agents, and cholesterol-lowering drugs. If you are using any of these medications, talk to your doctor prior to taking vitamin A.

Special considerations: Anyone with high cholesterol, heart disease, kidney disease, or at risk of osteoporosis should speak to his or her doctor before taking vitamin A. Don't take vitamin A if you have an intestinal malabsorption syndrome.

Vitamin B_1 (thiamin, thiamine)

The B vitamins are a group of diverse but interrelated nutrients that play critical metabolic roles. Of particular interest to asthmatics is that vitamin B deficiency is a factor in increased leukotrienes and prostaglandin E_2, key components of the asthma cascade. Vitamin B_1 is needed to make ATP, the energy molecule used by all cells, and is also necessary for carbohydrate, fat, and protein metabolism.

There is no research at the present time on B_1 supplements for asthma relief. The only asthma-relevant study reported that children who took the bronchodilator theophylline had low blood levels of vitamins B_1 and B_6.[7] However, there are no official recommendations for theophylline users to supplement their diet with B_1 or B_6. While it has been suggested that B_1 and B_6 supplementation may be beneficial to asthmatics taking theophylline, the scientific community is still evaluating the necessity of these supplements. From my perspective, considering that B_1 deficiency makes theophylline-induced seizures particularly severe, you may want to supplement your diet with thiamine while taking theophylline.

Dietary sources: Thiamine is found in beans, fish, peanuts, and meat.

Dosage: Most authorities recommend 10–25 mg of vitamin B_1 a day as part of a multivitamin or B-complex supplement.

Side effects: Side effects are rare and include low blood pressure, diarrhea, excess lung fluid, irritability, itching, nausea, sweating, throat tightness, and weakness.

Precautions during pregnancy: If you're pregnant or lactating, consult your physician before taking vitamin B_1 supplements.

Drug interactions: Interactions with diuretics, oral contraceptives, stavudine, and tricyclic antidepressants have been reported. If you are taking any of these medications, consult your doctor before taking thiamine.

Vitamin B_3 (inositol hexaniacinate, niacin, niacinamide, nicotinamide, nicotinic acid)

Niacin is used to treat alcohol withdrawal and high cholesterol. Necessary for carbohydrate and cholesterol metabolism, the value of vitamin B_3 in asthma is theoretical. Some authorities suspect that glucocorticoid resistance leads to steroid dependence in some asthmatics. Nicotinamide appears to be the "drug of choice" for reversing this resistance and may permit some asthmatics to reduce their steroid dose. Also of interest is one study indicating that B_3 blocks histamine release from mast cells.[8] Further supporting the benefit of niacin for asthma is a study indicating that nicotinamide diminished asthma symptoms and intensity of anaphylactic shock in rodents.[9] Additionally, the Second National Health and Nutrition Examination Survey (NHANES 2), a large population-based study of 9,074 adults, found that high dietary niacin reduced wheezing risk by 35 percent.[10] Another study indicated that nicotinamide may increase steroid production by the adrenal glands. When there is an increase in natural steroids, inflammation decreases, which for asthmatics translates into fewer symptoms.[11]

There has been only one trial to examine nicotinic acid supplementation for asthma. This study was published in Russia and combined vitamin B_3 with ascorbic acid (vitamin C). The authors reported that the combination helped asthmatics; however, since B_3 was given with vitamin C (known to benefit asthmatics), the results are inconclusive with respect to B_3. The authors also reported that niacin deficiency was common in asthmatics.[12] Nevertheless, further research is clearly needed. I have no objection to asthmatics taking niacin; if it doesn't help your asthma, it may lower your cholesterol.

Dietary sources: Vitamin B_3 is found naturally in brewer's yeast, fish, meat, and peanuts.

Dosage: Most people start with 100 mg of niacin daily and gradually increase their dose to 100–300 mg three times a day, taken with meals and at least two glasses of water. Do not take more than 1,000 mg of niacin a day without consulting a physician. Inositol hexaniacinate appears to be the safest form to use. Nevertheless, because safety studies are still pending, consult your physician before taking dosages over 2,000 mg a day.

Side effects: The most common side effect is flushing; however, headache, stomach pain, and vomiting can occur with dosages as low as 50 mg a day. Additional rare side effects can occur with higher dosages, including diabetes, diarrhea, dry skin, eye problems, gout, headache, irregular heart rhythms, liver toxicity, low blood pressure, muscle injury, nausea, skin rash, stomach pain or ulcers, and vomiting. Have your physician check for these side effects. Alcohol and hot drinks can increase niacin-associated flushing, whereas 125–350 mg of aspirin taken 20–30 minutes prior to taking niacin may prevent flushing.

Precautions during pregnancy: Some authorities recommend taking an additional 2 mg of niacin a day during pregnancy. If you are pregnant or lactating, speak to your doctor before taking a niacin supplement.

Drug interactions: Interactions are reported with atorvastatin, benztropine, carbidopa, fluvastatin, glimepiride, isoniazid, levodopa, lovastatin, minocycline, oral contraceptives, pravastatin, repaglinide, simvastatin, tetracycline, thioridazine, and tricyclic antidepressants. If you are using any of these medications, talk to your doctor before taking niacin.

Special considerations: Have your physician periodically check your blood and liver function while taking niacin. Do not use niacin if you have bleeding problems, liver disease, low blood pressure, or stomach ulcers. Finally, talk to your doctor prior to taking vitamin B_3 if you have diabetes, gallbladder disease, gout, jaundice, liver problems, heart disease, tartrazine sensitivity, or a history of stomach ulcers or bleeding.

Vitamin B_6 (pyridoxine, pyridoxal-5-phosphate, PLP)

Pyridoxine plays a critical role in the manufacture and breakdown of amino acids, the building blocks of proteins and hormones. Vitamin B_6 is also involved in neurotransmitter formation and is believed to play a role in how we think and feel. Along with vitamin B_{12} and folic acid, vitamin B_6 lowers homocysteine levels—which, when elevated, become a risk factor for heart disease. Pyridoxine is used in the treatment of several medical conditions, including acne, celiac disease, depression, diabetes, and premenstrual syndrome.

Vitamin B_6 is critical for normal processing of the neurotransmitter tryptophan, and researchers suspect that abnormal tryptophan metabolism plays a role in some asthmatics. One study found that pyridoxine levels were only 50 percent of normal in adults with asthma.[13] Depressed B_6 levels were also found in asthmatics taking theophylline, a common asthma medication.[14]

While there are only a few studies examining B_6 supplements and asthma, two trials have reported favorable results. One double-blind, controlled clinical trial studied seventy-six asthmatic children who took 200 mg of B_6 per day for five months. The researchers reported a significant improvement in asthma symptoms and a reduction in bronchodilator and cortisone dosage.[15] Another study involved seven asthmatics who supplemented with 50 mg of B_6 twice daily. While supplementation did not produce a sustained elevation in B_6 blood levels, the researchers did find that "all subjects reported a dramatic decrease in frequency and severity of wheezing or asthmatic attacks while taking the supplement."[16] A possible explanation for this benefit may be that B_6 blocks histamine release from mast cells.[17]

While these results are encouraging, a 1993 double-blind, placebo-controlled study failed to find any benefit in thirty-one steroid-dependent asthmatics who took 300 mg a day of pyridoxine.[18] These conflicting results may be related to study design, but considering the fact that only three studies exist, further investigation is warranted before any definitive recommendation can be made.

As for asthmatics who are taking theophylline, while it has been suggested that B_6 and B_1 supplementation may be beneficial, the scientific community is still evaluating the necessity of these supplements. Considering the negative role B_6 deficiency plays in theophylline-induced seizures, you may want to supplement with pyridoxine if you're using theophylline.

Dietary sources: Foods rich in B_6 include bananas, lentils, liver, potatoes, raisin bran, turkey, and tuna.

Dosage: Most authorities recommend 25–100 mg of B_6 once a day. If you're taking theophylline, 25–100 mg of vitamin B_6, daily, is recommended.

Side effects: Side effects are rare and usually occur only with doses over 200 mg a day. Numbness and trouble with walking are the most common side effects. Rare side effects include fatigue, headache, nausea, and poor coordination.

Precautions during pregnancy: Some authorities recommend an additional 0.6 mg of B_6 during pregnancy. Talk to your doctor if you are pregnant or lactating and thinking about taking a B_6 supplement.

Drug interactions: Interactions with antiseizure medications, barbiturates, carbidopa, corticosteroids, cycloserine, docetaxel, erythromycin, estrogens, fluorouracil, gentamicin, hydralazine, hydroxychloroquine, isoniazid, levodopa, neomycin, oral contraceptives, penicillamine, phenelzine, phenytoin, risperidone, steroids, sulfamethoxazole, tetracycline, and tricyclic antidepressants have been reported. If you are using any of these medications, talk to your doctor before taking B_6.

Special considerations: Speak to your doctor if you plan to take more than 100 mg of vitamin B_6 a day for longer than two months.

Folic Acid (folate, folinic acid, methylfolate)

Folic acid, a B vitamin, is involved in DNA and RNA synthesis. Playing a vital role in cellular reproduction and growth, folic acid also helps reduce homocysteine levels. The only established role folic acid deficiency has in asthma is for steroid-dependent asthmatics who use methotrexate, a drug that interferes with folic acid metabolism. Folic acid helps prevent many of the side effects associated with methotrexate use.

Dietary sources: Folic acid is found in beans, brewer's yeast, flour, grain products, lentils, meat, orange juice, rice, spinach, and leafy green vegetables.

Dosage: The typical recommended dose is 100–400 mcg of folic acid, daily; however, doses of 5,000 mcg a day are used by people taking methotrexate. Doses of 2,500–5,000 mcg of folinic acid may also be used. Doses over 1,000 mcg a day should not be taken without a doctor's permission. If you're using methotrexate, ask your physician what dose is right for you.

Side effects: No significant side effects have been reported. Rare side effects include bronchospasm, itching, and rash.

Precautions during pregnancy: Folic acid supplements are safe and encouraged during pregnancy to help prevent birth defects. Talk to your doctor about the correct dose for you.

Drug interactions: Interactions are reported with antacids, anti-seizure medications, aspirin, barbiturates, bile-acid sequestrants, cancer chemotherapy, colestipol, cycloserine, diuretics, erythromycin, famotidine, fluoxetine, indomethacin, isoniazid, lithium, medroxyprogesterone, metformin, methotrexate, neomycin, nitrous oxide, nizatidine, oral contraceptives, phenytoin, piroxicam, pyrimethamine, salsalate, sulfamethoxazole, sulindac, tetracycline, triamterene, and trimethoprim/sulfamethoxazole. If you are using any of these medications, check with your physician before taking folic acid.

Special considerations: Folic acid supplementation can delay the diagnosis of vitamin B_{12} deficiency. If you have a history of anemia, consult your doctor before taking folic acid.

Vitamin B_{12} (adenosylcobalamin, cobalamin, cyanocobalamin, hydroxocobalamin, hydroxycyanocobalamin, methylcobalamin)

Vitamin B_{12} is vital for normal nerve function and also helps reduce homocysteine, a protein that can increase the risk of heart disease. Cyanocobalamin deficiency is associated with fatigue, and B_{12} injections are sometimes used to treat chronic fatigue, depression, and pernicious anemia.

There has been only one study to evaluate B_{12} supplementation and asthma. It examined the effect of treating five sulfite-sensitive asthmatics with 1.5 mg of oral B_{12} prior to a sulfite challenge. As mentioned in Chapter 2, sulfites (commonly found in wine) can trigger an asthma attack in sensitive asthmatics. In four of the five patients, the sulfite sensitivity was abolished by pretreatment with cyanocobalamin. In three of these four patients, the blocking effect of B_{12} lasted from four to thirteen days.[19] More studies on B_{12} and asthma are clearly warranted; however, these results are intriguing for asthmatics who are wine lovers.

Dietary sources: Vitamin B_{12} is commonly found in meat, fish, and dairy products.

Dosage: Recommendations vary depending on the condition treated. Strict vegetarians usually require 2–3 mcg a day, whereas a dose of 1,000 mcg a day is standard for pernicious anemia. Some authorities recommend that the elderly take 10–25 mcg of B_{12} daily. As cobalamin deficiency is rare, most people do not need supplements.

Side effects: Side effects are rare with oral B_{12}; however, diarrhea and occasional allergic reactions to B_{12} injections may occur.

Precautions during pregnancy: If you are pregnant or lactating, talk to your doctor before taking a B_{12} supplement.

Drug interactions: Interactions are reported with antiseizure medications, AZT, cimetidine, clofibrate, colchicine, erythromycin, famotidine, isoniazid, lansoprazole, metformin, methyldopa, neomycin, nitrous oxide, nizatidine, omeprazole, oral contraceptives, ranitidine, sulfamethoxazole, tetracycline, and tricyclic antidepressants. If you use any of these medications, talk to your doctor before taking vitamin B_{12}.

Special considerations: Do not take vitamin B_{12} if you are allergic to cobalt.

Vitamin C (ascorbate, ascorbic acid)

Vitamin C is perhaps the most important vitamin for asthmatics. Not only is vitamin C the lung's chief free-radical scavenger, but it also protects the heart by preventing LDL-cholesterol oxidation, a risk factor for heart disease. Vitamin C is critical for building collagen, the connective tissue that holds our bodies together, and for wound healing. If you have allergies, you'll be happy to know that ascorbic acid also acts as an antihistamine. Vitamin C deficiency is linked to cancer, diabetes, heart disease, and asthma.

Vitamin C is absolutely critical for normal lung function and is the lung's leading antioxidant. Contained in the fluid that lines the lungs, vitamin C plays a pivotal role in protecting the lungs from oxidative stress and damage. Oxidant stress is blamed for many human ills, including asthma. Studies have shown that vitamin C can shift critical metabolic pathways from producing prostaglandin F_2, a bronchoconstrictor, to prostaglandin E_2, a bronchodilator.[20] It also plays a role in regenerating vitamin E, another powerful antioxidant. And there is evidence that vitamin C supplementation can reduce levels of histamine (a potent bronchoconstrictor) in the blood by up to 40 percent.[21]

There is an emerging consensus that low vitamin C intake is a risk factor for asthma.[22] Numerous researchers have documented that reduced dietary vitamin C is associated with lung disease, and large population studies have found that the less fruit consumed (lower vitamin C intake), the higher the incidence of asthma. Given these considerations, it should not be surprising to learn that low blood levels of vitamin C are found in adults and children with asthma. Studies show that, in asthmatics, the fluid that lines the lungs is deficient in vitamin C. That's bad news considering people with asthma have increased antioxidant demands, and vitamin C is critical to healthy lung function.

Vitamin C deficiency also appears to play a role in the shift from Th1 to Th2 T-cells, which results in increased leukotrienes and prostaglandin E_2, potent chemical mediators of the asthma cascade. Emotional, physical, and environmental stress factors are also known to lower vitamin C levels. Even worse, there is evidence that the leukocytes (white blood cells critical to proper immune function) of asthmatics are deficient in vitamin C.

Conversely, there are multiple studies indicating that high vitamin C intake can protect and help people with asthma. For asthma-allergy sufferers, there is even evidence that increased vitamin C intake reduces atopy, a major risk factor for asthma and allergies. Equally important, vitamin C can reduce the duration and severity of the common cold, a major cause of asthma exacerbations. There is also significant evidence indicating that vitamin C can jump-start the immune system and reduce IgE levels. IgE is an antibody and the prime mediator of the allergic response; elevated IgE is believed to correspond to asthma and allergy severity.

Perhaps the most important study of vitamin C and lung function came from the Environmental Protection Agency and reviewed over 2,500 adults as part of the First National Health and Nutrition Examination Survey (NHANES I). This study examined the effect of vitamin C on FEV_1, an important measure of lung function. The authors found that vitamin C had a protective effect on lung function and that low vitamin C intake was "directly related to lower values of FEV_1." The study concluded that vitamin C had a "fivefold greater protective effect" in asthma.[23] Supporting these findings was a 2001 study from Taiwan involving 1,166 teenagers, which also demonstrated that low vitamin C intake increased asthma risk.[24]

With respect to airway reactivity, one randomized, double-blind, placebo-controlled trial from Yale University demonstrated that vitamin C (500 mg four times a day for three days) completely prevented airway hyperresponsiveness to nitrogen dioxide, a known bronchoconstrictor.[25] Similar results have also been reported for ozone and methacholine (a bronchoconstrictor). Supporting the ability of ascorbate to reduce airway reactivity was another Yale study, which found that a gram of vitamin C reduced airway responsiveness to methacholine in asthmatics.[26] Finally, a cross-sectional study of 2,000 adults from Scotland reported that people who consumed low levels of vitamin C were four times more likely to have hyperactive airways compared to those with high vitamin C intake.[27]

One of the first studies to directly examine vitamin C supplements for asthmatics was conducted in Nigeria in 1980. In this randomized, placebo-controlled trial, scientists examined the effect of vitamin C (1,000 mg a day for fourteen weeks) in a group of forty-one asthmatics. At the end of the study, those taking ascorbic acid suffered less severe and less frequent asthma attacks. When the participants stopped taking ascorbic acid, the attack rates increased.[28]

Indirect evidence of the positive role ascorbic acid plays in asthma was offered by researchers at the Saint George's Hospital Medical School in London, who studied the impact of fresh fruit and vegetable consumption in 2,650 children. Researchers found that FEV_1 improved in asthmatic children who consumed a fruit-rich diet, with a similar but less dramatic improvement in FEV_1 for children who consumed green vegetables. The most significant impact of fresh fruit was observed in children who wheezed, suggesting that the mechanism of action is "protection against bronchoconstriction."[29]

Similar results have been reported by other studies. One Italian study of over 18,000 participants concluded that there was a clear association between low fruit intake and an increased risk of wheezing. Only 29.3 percent of subjects who consumed fruit at least once a week reported wheezing compared to 47.1 percent of those who ate fruit less than once a week.[30] A British study examined almost 3,000 adults and found that regular fruit consumption significantly improved FEV_1.[31] Finally, a 1999 study examined over 10,000 men and women and reported that "their findings support postulated associations between infrequent fresh fruit consumption and the prevalence of frequent or severe asthma symptoms in adults."[32]

Several studies have examined the impact of vitamin C on exercise-induced asthma (EIA). One randomized, placebo-controlled study pretreated twelve asthmatics with 500 mg of ascorbic acid and found that "pretreatment with ascorbic acid led to a significant attenuation of the bronchospasm seen five minutes after exercise compared to placebo."[33] Another study gave 2 grams of vitamin C or placebo to subjects prior to treadmill testing. Lung function was tested in both groups before and after exercise. Researchers found that vitamin C "prevented the development of EIA in nine of twenty patients and reduced the airways' responsiveness to exercise in two other patients."[34]

While light-to-moderate exercise may enhance the immune system, demanding events like marathons can temporarily depress immune function and lead to increased viral infections in athletes. Studies have documented that vitamin C can reduce the incidence of these infections. One trial supplemented ultramarathon runners with 600 mg of vitamin C, daily. The runners were followed for two weeks post-marathon; only 33 percent of the vitamin C group caught a cold, compared to 68 percent of the placebo group. Plus, the upper respiratory tract infections that did occur in the vitamin C group were significantly shorter in duration and less severe than in the control group.[35]

When all is said and done, we are seeing the emergence of a powerful body of literature documenting that, for many asthmatics, vitamin C can significantly improve symptoms. The reasons why vitamin C helps asthmatics are complex, but part of the explanation undoubtedly lies in the ability of vitamin C to enter the lungs and fight free radicals. Like any supplement or medication, vitamin C may work for one person but not for another; nevertheless, after reviewing the literature, vitamin C gets a big "thumbs-up" from me.

Dietary sources: Found in many fruits and vegetables, vitamin C is especially abundant in broccoli, Brussels sprouts, citrus fruits, currants, kiwifruit, parsley, red peppers, rose hips, and strawberries.

Dosage: Most people take 500–1,000 mg of vitamin C a day, divided into two to three doses.

Side effects: While many people can tolerate 2,000–4,000 mg of vitamin C a day, doses over 2,000 mg daily are not recommended and can cause nausea, stomach pain, diarrhea, kidney stones, and copper deficiency. Other side effects include dizziness, excessive urination, flushing, headache, heartburn, insomnia, and vomiting.

Precautions during pregnancy: If you are pregnant or lactating, speak to your doctor before taking vitamin C supplements.

Drug interactions: Interactions with acetaminophen (Tylenol), allopurinol, ampicillin, antibiotics, aspirin, cancer chemotherapy agents, carbidopa, Cardec, clozapine, corticosteroids, cyclophosphamide, doxorubicin, epinephrine, indomethacin, isosorbide mononitrate, levodopa, minocycline, nitroglycerine, Nitroglyn, oral contraceptives, perphenazine, salsalate, tacrine, tetracycline, thioridazine, and warfarin have been reported. If you are using any of these medications, talk to your doctor before taking vitamin C.

Special considerations: If you have a history of diabetes, kidney stones, kidney failure, glucose-6-phosphate dehydrogenase deficiency, gout, sulfite or tartrazine sensitivity, or have an iron overload problem (hemochromatosis or hemosiderosis), talk to your doctor before taking vitamin C. If you are using medications to thin your blood, you should also consult your doctor before taking vitamin C. Since vitamin C supplements can interfere with copper metabolism, it's important to take a multivitamin and mineral supplement containing copper.

Vitamin D (1,25-dihydroxyvitamin D, calciferol, calcipotriol, cholecalciferol or D_3, ergocalciferol or D_2)

Vitamin D is the calcium gatekeeper, making sure there is a healthy balance of calcium between the blood and bones. While calciferol is found in several "vitamin D fortified" foods, most vitamin D is made in the skin during exposure to sunlight. Used to treat rickets and Crohn's disease, vitamin D's only known benefit in asthma is to help prevent steroid-induced osteoporosis, one of the more dreaded and potentially debilitating side effects of corticosteroids. Research has, however, been conducted on vitamin D and asthma. One controlled clinical trial in 1976 examined the combined use of calcium and vitamin D_2 in twelve asthmatics. The authors reported "a statistically significant reduction of airway resistance as well as an increase in FEV_1."[36] This small study, however, obviously doesn't cut it; further research is needed to investigate this potential association.

Dietary sources: While most vitamin D is made by the body when the skin is exposed to sunlight, cod liver oil is a rich natural source of this vitamin. Small amounts of vitamin D are also found in butter and egg yolks, but loading up on these sources will not help your cholesterol. Many foods are fortified with vitamin D.

Dosage: Most people with average sunlight exposure do not need additional vitamin D. If, however, you are using steroids, the American College of Rheumatology recommends 250–500 IU of vitamin D with 800 mg of calcium, daily. An alternative treatment is 1 mcg of alfacalcidol or 0.5 mcg of calcitriol (active forms of vitamin D), daily, along with calcium. If you are not taking steroids, a dose of 400–1,000 IU a day is recommended for supplementation.

Side effects: Side effects include constipation, dry mouth, headaches, kidney stones, loss of appetite, nausea, stomach cramps, vomiting, and weight loss. Infrequent side effects include decreased sex drive, diarrhea, fatigue, hearing loss, hypertension, irregular heart rhythms, itching, mood changes (irritability), polydipsia (increased thirst), polyuria (increased urination), seizures, vision loss, weakness, and even death. These are rare side effects and virtually every report of vitamin D toxicity occurred with dosages over 40,000 IU a day.

Precautions during pregnancy: If you are lactating or are pregnant, consult your doctor prior to taking vitamin D supplements.

Drug interactions: Interactions with allopurinol, antiseizure medications, barbiturates, bile-acid sequestrants, cimetidine, colestipol, oral corticosteroids, estrogens, heparin, hydroxychloroquine, indapamide, isoniazid, medroxyprogesterone, mineral oil, neomycin, sodium fluoride, thiazide diuretics, verapamil, and warfarin have been reported. If you are using any of these drugs, talk to your doctor before taking vitamin D.

Special considerations: If you have a history of heart disease, hyperparathyroidism, kidney disease, sarcoidosis, or intend to take more than 1,000 IU of vitamin D a day, consult your doctor before using vitamin D. Do not take vitamin D if you have kidney failure or a history of elevated blood levels of calcium or phosphate.

Vitamin E (alpha-tocopherol, tocopherol, tocopheryl)

Vitamin E is a generic term for eight fat-soluble molecules, only one of which, alpha-tocopherol, is active in humans. The body's leading lipid antioxidant, vitamin E helps protect every organ and cell from oxidative damage. There is a substantive body of literature indicating that vitamin E protects against heart disease, high cholesterol, cancer, diabetes, cataracts, and macular degeneration. With respect to heart disease, a study published in *The New England Journal of Medicine* reported that people who took at least 100 IU of vitamin E daily for two years or more reduced their risk of heart disease by 37 percent for men and 41 percent for women.[37] Though a super antioxidant, vitamin E can't do the job alone and interacts synergistically with vitamin C, beta-carotene, selenium, and other nutrients to protect our bodies from oxidative stress.

Alpha-tocopherol deficiencies, like vitamin C deficiencies, are found in asthmatics, especially in the fluid that lines the lungs. In fact, several authorities suspect that low vitamin E may be a more potent risk factor for asthma than low vitamin C.[38] Vitamin E deficiency also appears to play a role in the shift from Th1 to Th2 T-cells, resulting in increased leukotrienes and prostaglandin E_2, mediators of the asthma cascade. Serious vitamin E deficiency is rare, however, and usually only found in people with liver disease or fat malabsorption.

Especially important to asthmatics is the role vitamins E and C play in enhancing immune function. One randomized, placebo-controlled trial from the USDA Human Nutrition Research Center on Aging, at Tufts University, examined vitamin E supplementation in eighty-eight individuals. After four months of administering 200 mg of vitamin E a day, investigators found that immune function increased 65 percent in the vitamin E group versus 17 percent in the placebo group.[39] In the Netherlands, similar but less dramatic results were reported in another group given 100 mg of vitamin E daily for six months.[40]

There is also evidence that vitamin E can improve lung function and reduce airway reactivity. In one study, combined administration of vitamins C and E inhibited ozone-induced bronchoconstriction.[41] Vitamin E deficiency may also be a risk factor for asthma. One study examined ninety-four asthmatics over thirty years and found that those with the lowest levels of vitamin E intake were four times more likely to experience wheezing.[42] Another study examined the impact of vitamin E on lung function and found that "for every milligram increase in vitamin E in the daily diet, FEV_1 increased by an estimated 42 ml and FVC by an estimated 54 ml," a significant improvement.[43]

Also like vitamin C, vitamin E may protect against asthma. One Harvard study of 77,866 women found that those who had the highest dietary intake of vitamin E cut their risk of asthma by almost 50 percent.[44] Further supporting the relationship between low tocopherol levels and asthma is a study demonstrating that brittle asthmatics had less dietary intake of vitamin E than healthy adults.[45]

For the allergic asthmatic, there is evidence that vitamin E limits the allergic response. IgE is a major allergy mediator and people with asthma and allergies often have elevated blood levels of IgE. A collaborative study conducted by Harvard and the University of Nottingham on 2,633 adults concluded that "higher concentrations of vitamin E intake were associated with lower serum IgE concentrations and a lower frequency of allergen sensitization." The study also found that increased vitamin E intake reduced atopy risk, airway hyperresponsiveness, hay fever, and asthma.[46]

How does vitamin E work its magic? In addition to acting as a potent free-radical scavenger, vitamin E inhibits leukotriene synthesis. Evidence suggests that tocopherol "strongly inhibits" the 5-lipooxygenase pathway, which leads to leukotriene synthesis and also blocks the activation of neutrophils, potent inflammatory cells that can increase leukotrienes. Leukotrienes play a pivotal role in the asthma cascade and are responsible for many asthma symptoms. Some of the most successful pharmaceuticals for asthma work by blocking leukotriene synthesis.

Given the substantial body of literature supporting the effectiveness of vitamins C and E as asthma fighters, vitamin E supplements earn my endorsement for people with allergies and asthma.

Dietary sources: Being a fat-soluble vitamin, natural alpha-tocopherol is found in fatty foods such as egg yolks, nuts, seeds, and vegetable oils (almond, sunflower, and wheat germ). Whole-grain cereals and leafy green vegetables are also good tocopherol sources.

Dosage: The typical vitamin E dosage is 400–800 IU daily; however, there is emerging evidence that daily dosages of 100–200 IU may be just as effective. Most studies use a daily dose of 100–800 IU, an intake that requires the consumption of a high-fat diet. Given this consideration, most people who wish to increase their vitamin E levels take supplements.

Natural vitamin E is the preferred supplement form. On a supplement label, "d-alpha-tocopherol" means the supplement is from a natural source. If you see "dl-alpha-tocopherol," the supplement is synthetic. Natural vitamin E is also called RRR-alpha-tocopherol, whereas the synthetic form may be called all-rac-alpha-tocopherol. To make things more complicated, synthetic vitamin E only comes in the alpha form, whereas natural vitamin E is available in the alpha form or mixed with beta, delta, and gamma forms. And just when you thought vitamin E could not get any more confusing, d-alpha-tocopherol comes in acetate and succinate forms that differ slightly in potency. All you really need to know is that natural vitamin E is more active and better absorbed than its synthetic counterpart and is the preferred supplement. Just remember, "d" is natural and "dl" is synthetic.

Side effects: Side effects are rare; they are usually seen with dosages over 1,000 IU a day. Potential side effects include abdominal pain, bleeding, blurred vision, diarrhea, fatigue, headache, hypertension, immune system dysfunction, nausea, stomach cramps, weakness, and glucose intolerance in people who are obese (glucose intolerance is a risk factor for diabetes).

Precautions during pregnancy: If you are pregnant or lactating, talk to your physician before taking vitamin E supplements.

Drug interactions: Interactions have been reported with allopurinol, amiodarone, anthralin, aspirin, AZT, Benzamycin, bile-acid sequestrants, cancer chemotherapy, colestipol, Coumadin, cyclophosphamide, cyclosporine, dapsone, doxorubicin, gemfibrozil, glyburide, griseofulvin, haloperidol, insulin, iron, isoniazid, lindane, mineral oil, risperidone, simvastatin, sodium fluoride, valproic acid, and warfarin. If you are using any of these medications, speak to your doctor before supplementing with vitamin E.

Special considerations: Vitamin E should not be taken with alcohol or iron pills, since alcohol decreases absorption and inorganic iron destroys vitamin E.

Calcium

Calcium is the most abundant of the body's minerals, with almost all calcium residing in the bones. Besides being vital for healthy bones and teeth, calcium plays a pivotal role in muscle contraction, nerve conduction, and blood clotting. Used to treat celiac disease, osteoporosis, and rickets, calcium-rich diets may also protect against colon polyps. The only known use for calcium in asthma is for the prevention of steroid-induced osteoporosis, one of the most dreaded and potentially debilitating side effects of corticosteroids.

Dietary sources: Most dietary calcium comes from dairy products; however, sardines, tofu, and leafy green vegetables are additional sources.

Dosage: Calcium citrate and calcium citrate/malate appear to have the best absorption rates. For people between the ages of nineteen and fifty, 1,000 mg of calcium per day is the RDA; for those over fifty-one, the RDA is 1,200 mg a day. Most people take 800–1,000 mg of calcium a day. Since vitamin D is necessary for calcium absorption, 400 IU of vitamin D is usually taken with calcium. A daily multivitamin and mineral supplement is also recommended, since calcium competes with other minerals for absorption. If you are using steroids, the American College of Rheumatology recommends 250–500 IU of vitamin D with 800 mg of calcium daily.

Side effects: The most common side effects are bloating, constipation, and gas. Other potential side effects include diarrhea, excessive thirst, headache, heartburn, loss of appetite, nausea, vomiting, and weakness. Rarely, kidney stones result from excessive calcium intake. Milk-alkali syndrome is another rare side effect that occurs when people combine a dairy-rich diet to calcium carbonate supplements.

Precautions during pregnancy: Supplementation is not recommended during pregnancy or lactation.

Drug interactions: Interactions have been reported with albuterol, alendronate, aluminum hydroxide, barbiturates, bile-acid sequestrants, caffeine, calcium channel-blockers, calcitonin, ciprofloxacin, cisplatin, corticosteroids (inhaled and oral), cycloserine, diclofenac, digoxin, digitoxin, doxycycline, erythromycin, estrogen, felodipine, gentamicin, hydroxychloroquine, indapamide, indomethacin, iron, isoniazid, itraconazole, lactase, losartan, mineral oil, minocycline, nadolol, neomycin, ofloxacin, oral contraceptives, quinidine, sodium fluoride, sodium polystyrene sulfonate, steroids, sucralfate, sulfamethoxazole, Synthroid, tetracycline, thiazides, thyroid hormones, tobramycin, triamterene, and verapamil. If you use any of these medications, talk to your doctor before taking calcium.

Special considerations: Do not take calcium supplements without your physician's permission if you have parathyroid disease or kidney problems. Calcium should not be taken by people with bone tumors, digoxin toxicity, kidney failure, kidney stones, hyperparathyroidism, sarcoidosis, ventricular fibrillation, or a history of elevated calcium blood levels or calcium in the urine. Also, do not take calcium if you are dehydrated, on a fluid-restricted diet, or have a history of decreased bowel motility or bowel obstruction.

Copper

Necessary for iron absorption and metabolism, copper is a vital part of the antioxidant enzyme superoxide dismutase. Studies have shown reduced superoxide dismutase activity in asthma.[47] Also used to make ATP, the body's energy molecule, copper plays a critical role in collagen synthesis.

Unlike the vitamin and mineral deficiencies so common in asthmatics, *elevated* blood levels of copper have been associated with asthma. The Second National Health and Nutrition Examination Survey (NHANES 2), a large population-based study of 9,074 adults, reported that high blood levels of copper increased wheezing risk.[48] Confusing matters is a Harvard study that found the higher the copper concentration in drinking water, the higher the FEV and FEV_1.[49] This finding prompted researchers to speculate that copper deficiency may be related to poor lung function—a controversial hypothesis since high blood levels of copper appear to increase rather than decrease asthma risk. While these studies are intriguing, further research is clearly needed to determine the exact relationship between copper and asthma. Until this controversy is resolved, the only role copper has in asthma is for those individuals that take zinc, a mineral that interferes with copper absorption.

Dietary sources: Excellent sources of copper include cereals, meat, nuts, oysters, potatoes, and vegetables.

Dosage: Most authorities recommend 1–3 mg of copper a day, especially for people that use zinc. If you decide to take a supplement, use alkaline copper carbonate, copper sulfate, or cupric acetate, which tend to be better absorbed than cupric oxide.

Side effects: Rare side effects are usually only seen in high doses and include anemia, muscle pain, nausea, stomach pain, and vomiting.

Precautions during pregnancy: Most pregnant women do not need copper supplements. If you are pregnant or lactating, speak to your physician before taking a copper supplement.

Drug interactions: Interactions are reported with antacids, AZT, ciprofloxacin, etodolac, famotidine, ibuprofen, nabumetone, nizatidine, oral contraceptives, oxaprozin, penicillamine, and valproic acid. If you are using any of these medications, check with your physician before taking copper.

Special considerations: If you have new copper piping in your home, speak to your doctor before supplementing, because you may be absorbing copper from your drinking water. Don't take copper if you have Wilson's disease, a condition caused by excess copper.

Manganese

Manganese is an essential trace mineral used by antioxidant enzymes such as superoxide dismutase. As with copper, studies show that manganese superoxide dismutase activity is decreased in asthmatics.[50] Manganese is vital for the production of normal bone, cartilage, and skin. There is only one study relating manganese deficiency to asthma: a cross-sectional survey of 2,000 adults in England. Researchers found that individuals with the lowest intake of manganese had over eight times the risk of bronchial reactivity.[51] These impressive results point an accusing finger at manganese deficiency, but additional studies are clearly needed to confirm the role this deficiency plays in asthma.

Dietary sources: Manganese is found in nuts, pineapples, seeds, wheat bran, wheat germ, and leafy green vegetables.

Dosage: Most authorities recommend 2–5 mg a day; however, many multivitamin and mineral supplements contain up to 15 mg of manganese. Manganese deficiency may occur in people who take calcium, iron, or zinc, as these minerals can interfere with manganese absorption. Consider taking manganese or a multivitamin and mineral if you are using any of these supplements.

Side effects: Rare side effects are usually seen only with high doses and include dementia and other psychiatric problems.

Precautions during pregnancy: Most pregnant women do not need manganese supplements. Speak to your physician if you are considering taking manganese supplements while pregnant or lactating.

Drug interactions: Interactions are reported with ciprofloxacin and oral contraceptives. If you are using these medications, speak to your doctor before taking manganese.

Special considerations: People with liver disease or cirrhosis should not take manganese.

Magnesium

Magnesium is needed for just about everything, particularly to make bone, proteins, and ATP (energy molecules). Magnesium is also used to activate the B vitamins and to treat heart failure and irregular heart rhythms. As discussed earlier, the airways are surrounded by smooth muscles that contract during an asthma attack. A powerful smooth-muscle relaxant, magnesium was once used intravenously to treat severe asthma attacks.

Magnesium deficiency is reported in asthmatics, and it appears that the more severe the deficiency, the worse the asthma. Magnesium deficiency has also been linked to airway hyperreactivity. One study reported that the rate of hospitalization was 40 percent in asthmatics with magnesium deficiency compared to 12 percent in asthmatics with normal magnesium levels.[52] Researchers have found that, in asthmatics, magnesium deficiency is in part responsible for the increased airway response to irritants like methacholine. One study concluded that "the levels of intracellular magnesium are directly and strongly related to the reactivity of the bronchial airway."[53] Another trial demonstrated that low magnesium intake was associated with a fivefold increased risk of bronchial hyperreactivity.[54] Finally, a British study reported reduced dietary magnesium in brittle asthmatics. [55]

Not surprisingly, published reports indicate that magnesium improves lung function, reduces asthma symptoms, and protects against asthma. One study involving 2,633 adults found that high dietary magnesium increased FEV_1 while reducing airway reactivity and wheezing episodes.[56] Another study supplemented asthmatics with 400 mg of magnesium per day and reported a subsequent reduction in asthma symptoms. This study also found that, for people with high magnesium intake, the risk of airway reactivity was slashed in half.[57]

Magnesium helps asthmatics by relaxing bronchial smooth muscle and making the airways less reactive. There is also evidence that magnesium stabilizes mast cells and T lymphocytes, major cellular mediators of an asthma attack. Given the rapidly accumulating body of literature supporting the use of magnesium in asthma, magnesium supplements are strongly recommended.

Dietary sources: Magnesium is found in beans, cereals, dairy products, fish, meat, nuts, and dark green vegetables.

Dosage: Recommended daily intake of magnesium ranges from 240–420 mg and increases with age. The typical recommended supplement is 250–350 mg of magnesium a day. Since vitamin B_6 helps in magnesium absorption, many people take 10–25 mg of pyridoxine with magnesium. A daily multivitamin and mineral supplement is also recommended, since magnesium competes with other minerals for absorption.

Side effects: The most common side effect of magnesium is diarrhea. Rare side effects include burping, depression, excess gas, lethargy, nausea, stomach cramps, vomiting, and weakness.

Precautions during pregnancy: If you're pregnant or lactating, speak to your doctor before taking magnesium.

Drug interactions: Interactions have been reported with albuterol, alendronate, allopurinol, amiloride, amphotericin, aspirin, atenolol, azithromycin, cefpodoxime, cimetidine, ciprofloxacin, cisplatin, corticosteroids (oral), cycloserine, digoxin, diuretics, docusate, doxycycline, epinephrine, erythromycin, estrogens, famotidine, felodipine, gentamicin, glimepiride, glipizide, glyburide, hydroxychloroquine, iron, isoniazid, ketoconazole, levofloxacin, lomefloxacin, losartan, medroxyprogesterone, metformin, minocycline, misoprostol, neomycin, nitrofurantoin, nizatidine, norfloxacin, ofloxacin, oral contraceptives, pefloxacin, penicillamine, quinidine, sodium polystyrene sulfonate, spironolactone, sulfamethoxazole, tetracycline, tobramycin, and warfarin. If you are using any of these medications, talk to your doctor before taking magnesium.

Special considerations: If you have kidney problems, consult your doctor before taking magnesium. Do not take magnesium if you have diarrhea or a history of high blood levels of magnesium.

Selenium

King of the antioxidant minerals, selenium works synergistically with vitamin E to protect the heart and lungs from disease. Selenium also fights cancer by activating glutathione peroxidase, a potent antioxidant enzyme. One study reported that people who took 200 mcg of selenium for an average of 4.5 years reduced their cancer risk by 50 percent.[58] Especially important for asthmatics, selenium is vital for a healthy immune system. Selenium deficiency also appears to play a role in the shift from Th1 to Th2 T-cells, which increases levels of leukotrienes and prostaglandin E_2, mediators of the asthma cascade. Selenium deficiency is linked to asthma, arthritis, cancer, cataracts, and heart disease.

In studies, selenium deficiency has been found in asthmatics. A living laboratory that reflects the vital role selenium plays in asthma is New Zealand, where selenium-poor soil translates into low dietary selenium and a high prevalence of asthma. One study of fifty-six asthmatic and fifty-nine non-asthmatic subjects from New Zealand found that people with the lowest selenium levels had as much as 5.8 times the risk of asthma.[59] A randomized, placebo-controlled trial from Sweden, involving twenty-four asthmatics who received selenium daily for fourteen weeks, reported significant clinical improvement.[60] Another study from King's College in London, involving 9,709 individuals, found that high selenium intake reduced asthma risk by up to 25 percent.[61] Further supporting the relationship between selenium deficiency and asthma is the fact that brittle asthmatics tend to have reduced dietary selenium.[62]

While there is little doubt that selenium deficiency is an asthma risk factor, it remains to be determined whether selenium supplements can help asthmatics. Initial findings are promising, but additional studies are needed before a definitive recommendation can be made. Nevertheless, selenium's role as a potent antioxidant and potential asthma fighter makes supplementation a worthwhile endeavor.

Dietary sources: Dietary selenium intake depends in part on where the food you eat is grown, as some regions of the United States have selenium-poor soil. However, since food is transported throughout the country, getting enough dietary selenium is rarely, if ever, a problem. The most important dietary sources of selenium are Brazil nuts, grains, plant products, seafood, organ meats, and yeast.

Dosage: The typical recommended dose of selenium is 200 mcg a day.

Side effects: Side effects like selenosis (characterized by dry hair, fatigue, and irritability) usually occur with doses over 600 mcg a day. Other side effects include fingernail loss, nervous system problems, and skin rash. Severe selenium toxicity manifests as hair loss, nausea, skin depigmentation, tooth cavities, and vomiting.

Precautions during pregnancy: If you are pregnant or lactating, speak to your doctor before taking selenium supplements.

Drug interactions: Interactions have been reported with cisplatin, clozapine, and valproic acid. If you are using any of these medications, speak to your doctor before taking selenium.

Special considerations: If you have thyroid problems or a goiter, consult your doctor before using selenium supplements.

Zinc

Zinc is important for wound healing, fertility, and protein synthesis. Asthmatics will be especially pleased to learn that zinc boosts immune function, acts as an antioxidant, and may shorten the duration of the common cold. There is also increasing evidence that zinc plays a protective role in a number of diseases, including asthma, allergies, atherosclerosis, cancer, and AIDS.

It is theorized that zinc deficiency leads to altered immune function, which creates a favorable environment for asthma. Like many of the nutrient deficiencies we have discussed, zinc deficiency appears to play a role in the shift from Th1 to Th2 T-cells. Zinc is a vital component of the antioxidant enzyme superoxide dismutase, and studies show that superoxide dismutase activity is decreased in asthmatics.[63] We also know that zinc deficiency results in a considerable increase in the number of mast cells and plays a major role in allergies. One cross-sectional survey of 2,000 adults from England found that low zinc intake resulted in an increased risk of bronchial hyperreactivity.[64]

While zinc deficiency may play a role in asthma, further research is needed before we can definitively say that zinc supplements will help asthmatics. Nevertheless, given it's role an as antioxidant and immune booster, zinc supplementation may provide benefit.

Dietary sources: Zinc is found in black-eyed peas, eggs, fish, meat, oysters, tofu, and wheat germ.

Dosage: Most people who supplement with zinc take 15 mg a day, with food. If you intend to treat a cold with zinc, use zinc gluconate lozenges, as these appear to be the most effective. There are also zinc-based nasal gels such as Zicam that have been used successfully to treat the common cold. Since zinc interferes with copper absorption, take extra copper when supplementing with zinc (check that your zinc supplement doesn't already contain copper before purchasing a separate copper supplement). A daily multivitamin and mineral supplement is also recommended, since zinc competes with other minerals for absorption.

Side effects: Side effects are rare and are usually reported with lozenges, which can cause mouth pain, nausea, stomach pain, and vomiting. Demonstrating that there can be too much of a good thing, zinc dosages over 300 mg a day may actually suppress immune function.

Precautions during pregnancy: If you are pregnant or lactating, talk to your doctor prior to taking zinc supplements.

Drug interactions: Drug interactions have been reported with angiotensin-converting enzyme inhibitors (ACE inhibitors), aspirin, AZT, benazepril, Benzamycin, bile-acid sequestrants, cancer chemotherapy agents, captopril, chlorhexidine, ciprofloxacin, clindamycin (topical only), corticosteroids (oral and topical), doxycycline, enoxacin, estrogen, lisinopril, medroxyprogesterone, methyltestosterone, metronidazole (vaginal), minocycline, norfloxacin, ofloxacin, oral contraceptives, penicillamine, quinapril, ramipril, sodium fluoride, tetracycline, thiazide diuretics, valproic acid, and warfarin. If you are using any of these medications, talk to your doctor before taking zinc.

Thymus Gland Extract (thymomodulin)

Thymus gland extract is not a vitamin or mineral, but it may nonetheless help people with allergies and asthma. The thymus gland is located in the lower part of the neck and is intimately involved in immune function. There are two basic types of immune response: antibody-mediated and cell-mediated. Cell-mediated immunity plays a critical role in protecting our bodies against disease caused by bacteria, parasites, yeast, viruses, and allergies. The thymus gland is the chief regulator of cell-mediated immunity. Thymus gland extracts are commercially available and used to treat a variety of ailments, including the common cold. These extracts work by restoring proper immune function specifically by normalizing the CD4+ to CD8+ cell ratio, cells that participate in many immune reactions.

One Italian trial on subjects with a variety of illnesses, including atopic dermatitis, found that thymomodulin was effective in "correcting altered immunological parameters."[65] Researchers have also discovered that thymomodulin improves clinical symptoms and reduces the frequency of acute allergic episodes in people with allergic rhinitis and atopic dermatitis.[66] Another study examined the impact of daily thymomodulin (120 mg for four months) in twenty individuals with allergic rhinitis. According to the authors, thymomodulin reduced the number of allergic episodes and symptoms, and normalized IgE.[67]

With respect to asthma, a 1989 study found that thymomodulin significantly reduced airway responsiveness to methacholine (an airway constrictor) in patients with allergic asthma.[68] Another study examined thymomodulin in forty-one children with asthma and reported a significant reduction in asthmatic attacks as well as decreased IgE.[69]

Presently, the best evidence regarding thymus gland extracts relates to people with allergies; further research examining how this extract may help asthmatics is still needed. Nevertheless, given the substantial body of literature supporting the use of thymus gland extracts for allergies, a trial of this supplement is recommended for individuals who suffer from allergic asthma.

Dosage: Thymomodulin is not presently available in the United

States; however, a variety of other thymus gland extracts are available. Dosage depends on the manufacturer's directions.

Side effects: No significant side effects are reported with thymus gland extracts.

Precautions during pregnancy: If you are pregnant or lactating, talk to your doctor before taking thymus gland extracts.

Drug interactions: Drug interactions have been reported with cisplatin, cyclophosphamide, docetaxel, fluorouracil, interferon, and paclitaxel. If you are using any of these medications, speak to your physician before taking thymus gland extract.

A FINAL WORD ON SUPPLEMENTS

Nutritional supplements are potentially confusing, and choosing the right supplement is often a matter of trial and error. Because vitamins and minerals work best when taken together, a multivitamin and mineral supplement goes a long way toward protecting your health. No matter how healthy or ill you are, I strongly recommend taking a multivitamin and mineral supplement. There are many excellent supplements on the market, and I suggest you take one that meets, or preferably exceeds, the minimum recommended dietary allowances. The nice thing about multivitamin and mineral supplements is that you cover all your bases, achieving the greatest benefit with minimal effort.

If you decide to take an individual supplement, carefully review with a physician or a pharmacist all the prescription and nonprescription drugs you are using. While most vitamin and mineral supplements are safe when used as directed, the potential for drug interactions cannot be ignored. If you can't decide which supplement is right for you, enlist the aid of a trusted healthcare professional who can help you make a decision.

Supplements have the potential to help people who suffer from asthma. There is no substitute, however, for healthy living; supplements are only a small part of the overall health picture. The battle against asthma has many fronts, including diet, exercise, environmental controls, proper sleep habits, medications, supplements, and a positive mental attitude. But do not be lulled into believing that a pill is going to solve your health problems. Supplements can certainly play an important role in asthma relief; however, they must be incorporated into a larger plan of healthy living that protects the entire body.

chapter 8

Herbs for Asthma Relief

MANY OF THE DRUGS WE USE to treat illness literally have their roots in the plant kingdom. Herbs (or botanicals) contain molecules that, when purified, we call a drug. So, it is important to treat herbs with the same respect—and caution—as our most powerful pharmaceuticals.

Through millions of years of trial and error, civilization has found that certain plants have medicinal properties. Only since the emergence of modern chemistry have we been able to isolate and synthesize the natural magic our ancestors discovered. But what do we really mean when we say something is "natural" versus "synthetic"? From a purist perspective, we could say that the only "natural" products are those that are used as they are found in nature. With respect to botanicals, this means ingesting or applying the unaltered, raw plant product. We may place this botanical in a pill or drink it as a tea, but the herb remains fundamentally unchanged. In contrast, the word "synthetic," in conventional usage, means any material not found in nature. These definitions approximate the meanings of these complex and occasionally controversial words. Most people would agree that plastics are synthetic, since they do not occur in nature and only result from the manipulations of science. With respect to medicinal herbs, however, the line between natural and synthetic is less clear.

For example, ephedrine can be obtained naturally from the plant *Ephedra sinica* or in synthesized form. Both products contain an identical chemical we call "ephedrine," with the only difference being that one is made in a laboratory and the other is found in a plant. Fundamentally, whether or not your ephedrine comes from a plant or a lab, they both contain the same active agent, ephedrine. The ephedrine you get from the lab has the same molecular structure as the ephedrine you get from a plant. This is, however, where the similarities end and the differences begin.

The choice between natural and synthetic is often a double-edged sword. A potential problem with some herbal preparations is that, unless the formulation is standardized, the consumer can never be sure how much active ingredient he or she is taking. This is usually not a problem with isolated or synthesized medications, for which strict formulary standards exist. The downside to modern pharmaceuticals is that they often contain additives, like preservatives and colorings, that can spell trouble for an asthmatic. This is a problem you don't usually see with herbs.

Another potential problem with herbal remedies, especially herbal combinations, is that they may contain additional active ingredients that you don't need or that could be dangerous. With pharmaceuticals, you know what you're getting; they may contain preservatives and colorings, but you can read about them on the label.

HERBS VS. PHARMACEUTICALS

Humans seek predictability, a need that is especially acute for things we ingest. Though we rarely speak about it, it's comforting to know that a cold glass of water will always taste like a cold glass of water and never burn our tongue. We demand the same predictability from the medicines we take, and we have a strong need to know the risks associated with the pills we swallow. Before we were able to analyze and synthesize medications, we were stuck with what we had. Through experience, we knew what to expect from a particular medicinal herb. However, if that agent had an undesirable side effect, we either didn't take it, accepted the side effect as a part of treatment, or used another botanical.

As technology advanced, we isolated the active ingredients behind these medicinal herbs and were able to synthesize and ultimately manipulate these molecules, often enhancing their therapeutic benefit and eliminating side effects. Molecular biology and organic chemistry also permitted us to develop agents not found in nature, agents that were often more potent than their herbal ancestors. Through standardized testing mandated by agencies like the US Food and Drug Administration, we know what to expect from the majority of pharmaceuticals. In other words, technology and the scientific method allow us to increase dramatically the predictability of the agents we use to treat illness. While it is true that we cannot predict with absolute certainty how a particular individual will react to a given pharmaceutical, through the process of standardized trials we have a good idea of what to expect.

The downside to synthesized pharmaceuticals is that they can result in toxic waste products that are harmful to the environment. From an economic perspective, the manufacturing of new drugs permits pharmaceutical companies to patent and occasionally charge exorbitant fees for their products. On the flip side, synthesis has dramatically reduced the economic and environmental costs of some drugs. Nevertheless, there are and probably always will be problems with the way we make and market pharmaceuticals.

I will not deny that much of the resistance of conventional medicine to integrative therapies stems from arrogance and a desire to discourage competition. There are, however, two sides to every story, and while the pharmaceutical industry is far from perfect, many people would not be alive today if it were not for modern drugs.

Minerals, herbs, and vitamins, like pharmaceuticals, are big business. Integrative therapies and their associated products represent a multibillion-dollar industry. And like the pharmaceutical companies, the herbal industry has its strengths and weaknesses. Medicinal herbs frequently offer consumers products that are not available elsewhere, products that are usually preservative- and additive-free—an important consideration for sensitive asthmatics. However, one of the greatest challenges faced by the herbal industry is standardization. Overall, the herbal industry lacks standardized formulations, so that consumers cannot always be sure how much active ingredient they are ingesting. This lack of standardization upsets the human need for predictability and is the leading reason why some people believe that herbs, just like other food or drug products, need federal oversight. While the vast majority of herbal manufacturers are responsible, there are reports of adulterated and mislabeled products finding their way into the market.

As for efficacy, we are beginning to see the publication of rigorous studies on herbal products in respected medical journals. While these studies are encouraging, documenting efficacy will take years of research and controversy. Finally, while pharmaceuticals can have a devastating impact on the environment, so too can herbs. For instance, the herb goldenseal (*Hydrastis canadensis*) is endangered because it is overharvested for its medicinal properties. While the herbal industry is far from perfect, think about all the lives herbs have saved through the millennia.

This is the balanced approach to integrative and conventional medicine that I would like to share with you. Keep in mind that the herb that works for one person may not work for you and that some people are even allergic to botanicals. Nevertheless, despite their potential shortcomings, herbs can help asthmatics. Like vitamins and minerals, combined herbal formulations tend to work better than single herbs, a phenomenon herbalists call "orchestration" or "creating a symphony." If you decide to take herbs, I suggest you do so under the guidance of a healthcare professional familiar with herbal therapy. Remember, the line between herb and drug is at best blurred, and many a powerful drug had a humble beginning as a "weed" in somebody's backyard.

BOSWELLIA SERRATA (FRANKINCENSE, SALAI GUGGAL)

Type: Traditional Indian (Ayurvedic) herbal medicine

Uses: Arthritis and ulcerative colitis

Active ingredient: Boswellic acids

Mechanisms of action: Inhibits leukotriene synthesis with attendant anti-inflammatory properties

A tree indigenous to India, *Boswellia serrata* contains a resin that has been used for centuries to treat painful conditions such as osteoarthritis, bursitis, and rheumatoid arthritis. Of interest to asthmatics, the resin contains boswellic acids, which limit leukotriene synthesis and have anti-inflammatory properties. Leukotrienes are potent mediators of the asthma cascade. Several pharmacologic agents work by blocking leukotriene synthesis.

One double-blind, placebo-controlled study looked at forty asthmatics who used 300 mg of *Boswellia* extract three times a day. After six weeks, 70 percent of the *Boswellia* group reported a reduction in or "disappearance" of wheezing and shortness of breath. The authors also reported a decrease in eosinophils and an increase in FEV_1 following *Boswellia* therapy. Only 27 percent of the placebo group reported improved asthma symptoms.[1] Since there has been only one controlled study, additional research is needed to establish the efficacy of *Boswellia* in fighting asthma. Results, however, are encouraging and, given the relative lack of side effects, *Boswellia* extract is worth trying.

Dosage: A typical dose is 150–400 mg of standardized extract, three times a day, for six to twelve weeks. The exact dosage depends on the percentage of boswellic acids in the extract, and the duration of treatment depends on symptoms. Optimal *Boswellia* dosage for asthma remains to be determined. Most extracts contain 37.5 to 65 percent boswellic acids.

Side effects: Side effects are rare but may include diarrhea, nausea, and rash.

Precautions during pregnancy: No definitive studies or guidelines could be found, so the use of *Boswellia* during pregnancy or lactation is not recommended.

Drug interactions: There are no reported drug interactions with *Boswellia.*

EPHEDRA SINICA (EPHEDRINE, MA HUANG, DESERT HERB, DESERT TEA, MORMON TEA)

Type: Traditional Chinese medicine

Uses: Allergies, asthma, cough, and weight loss

Active ingredients: Ephedrine and pseudoephedrine alkaloids

Mechanisms of action: Central nervous system stimulant and anti-inflammatory that inhibits prostaglandin E_2 synthesis

A Chinese shrub that has been used medicinally for over 5,000 years, *Ephedra sinica* is a natural source of ephedrine, a common ingredient in asthma, allergy, and cough preparations. While the *Ephedra* shrub is found in many desert climates, it is the Asian species that is medicinally active through the alkaloids ephedrine and pseudoephedrine. First isolated in 1887, ephedrine is a central nervous system stimulant that has also been used for weight loss. For asthmatics, the chief benefits of ephedrine are its anti-inflammatory activity and its ability to inhibit prostaglandin E_2 synthesis, which contributes to bronchodilation.

While the effects of pharmaceutical ephedrine on asthma are well-known, research examining herbal *Ephedra* in asthmatics is scant. One study from China reported that a liquid ma huang preparation improved asthma symptoms and lowered IgE levels; however, lack of pertinent data prevents a critical review of these findings.[2] *Ephedra sinica* is also used in several herbal preparations, including one called Strengthening Body Resistance Method (SBR) that, according to one Chinese study, markedly increased FEV_1.[3]

While ephedrine's efficacy as a bronchodilator is well documented, there are no randomly controlled trials examining herbal *Ephedra* in North America or Europe. Three encouraging Chinese studies exist, but their results need to be validated. Given these considerations, a strong recommendation for *Ephedra sinica* would be premature; however, asthmatics may cautiously consider herbal *Ephedra* as a possible alternative to ephedrine, but only under the guidance of a healthcare professional familiar with herbal therapies.

Dosage: According to the *Physicians' Desk Reference,* the average single dose is 15–30 mg of ephedrine, for a total dose of 300 mg per day. Using powdered stems that contain less than 1 percent ephedrine, 1.5–4 grams per day is often recommended as a tea, divided into two to three doses. Tinctures are also available (1–4 ml three times a day). Long-term use of *Ephedra* is not recommended.

Side effects: *Ephedra* is a stimulant and, if abused, can have amphetaminelike side effects that include anxiety, dry mouth, increased heart rate, headache, hypertension, insomnia, irregular heart rhythm, muscle restlessness, nausea, vomiting, urinary problems, and even death. *Ephedra* is potentially addictive and, if used for extended periods, can cause kidney stones. Poisoning occurs in high dosages with the following symptoms: asphyxiation, blood-chemistry disturbances, fever, heart failure, large pupils, muscle spasms, and sweating.

Precautions during pregnancy: Do not use *Ephedra* if you are pregnant or lactating.

Drug interactions: Interactions have been reported with caffeine, Cardec DM, corticosteroids, digitoxin, digoxin, epinephrine, glycosides, guanethidine, halothane, nadolol, oxytocin, phenelzine, phenylpropanolamine, secale alkaloid derivatives, and MAO inhibitors (antidepressants). If you are using any of these medications, talk to your doctor before taking *Ephedra sinica* or ephedrine.

Contraindications: *Ephedra* is contraindicated in people with hypertension, hyperthyroidism, glaucoma, nervous/anxiety disorders, prostate problems (difficulty urinating), or an adrenal gland tumor (pheochromocytoma). Do not use *Ephedra* without a doctor's permission if you have diabetes or heart disease.

Special considerations: Since *Ephedra* can suppress adrenal gland function, you'll need to take vitamin B_6, vitamin C, magnesium, and pantothenic acid supplements if you intend to use *Ephedra* for an extended period of time. Pseudoephedrine can make you sleepy, so avoid driving or performing potentially hazardous activities, such as operating heavy machinery, when using *Ephedra.* When storing *Ephedra sinica,* it must be protected from light.

GINKGO BILOBA (MAIDENHAIR TREE)

Type: Traditional Chinese medicine

Uses: Alzheimer's disease, atherosclerosis, and depression

Active ingredient: Ginkgo flavone glycosides and terpene lactones

Mechanism of action: Anti-inflammatory and antioxidant

Found indigenously in the United States, China, and France, ginkgo trees can live as long as 1,000 years. The plant has a noble 5,000-year history of use in treating memory loss, erectile dysfunction, and atherosclerosis.

With respect to asthma, studies show that ginkgo extracts limit or entirely prevent anaphylactic bronchoconstriction in animals.[4] Ginkgo extracts also inhibit platelet-activating factor, an important mediator of the asthma cascade. Other studies have shown that ginkgo reduces inflammation and blocks histamine-induced bronchoconstriction in mammals.[5] In one randomized, controlled clinical trial, sixty-one asthmatics were given ginkgo leaf liquor three times a day. This study reported a 10 percent increase in FEV_1 after four weeks, which rose to 15 percent after eight weeks. According to the authors, ginkgo "significantly reduced airway hyperreactivity and improved clinical symptoms."[6] Like many herbal remedies, controlled scientific studies are still limited; however, given the rare incidence of side effects with *Ginkgo biloba,* this herb is worth a try for asthmatics seeking an herbal therapy.

Dosage: The most common dose is 60–80 mg, two to three times a day, of standardized extract (containing 24 percent flavone glycosides and 6 percent terpene lactones).

Side effects: Side effects are rare and include headache and stomach upset.

Precautions during pregnancy: Speak to your physician before taking ginkgo if you are pregnant or lactating.

Drug interactions: Interactions have been reported with aspirin, citalopram, cyclosporine, diuretics, fluoxetine, fluvoxamine, heparin, paroxetine, sertraline, ticlopidine, trazodone, and warfarin. If you are using any of these medications, speak to your doctor before taking *Ginkgo biloba.*

Special considerations: Effects may take up to eight weeks to manifest. Protect ginkgo from light and moisture during storage.

HEDERA HELIX (GUM IVY, IVY LEAF, TRUE IVY, WOODBIND)

Type: Traditional Japanese (Kampo) herbal medicine

Uses: Asthma, bronchitis, cough, and stretch marks

Active ingredients: Saponins that prevent bronchoconstriction

Mechanisms of action: Expectorant and possible bronchodilator

Native to Europe, ivy is a climbing plant that decorates many walls and gardens. The Greeks believed a crown of ivy offered protection against the negative effects of alcohol, a tradition practiced even today during fraternity parties. Besides being an antispasmodic and expectorant, ivy extract is purported to exert antibacterial, antifungal, antiprotozoic, and antihelminthic actions.

One study from Germany examined the effects of ivy leaf extract on asthma. This double-blind, randomized, crossover trial involved twenty-four asthmatic children who took 35 mg of dried ivy leaf extract for three days. The authors reported that the extract decreased airway resistance by 23.6 percent but did not significantly improve FEV_1.[7] While this study is promising, more extensive trials will be needed before a definitive conclusion can be reached. Until that time, it can be reasonably said that ivy leaf extract appears to help some people with asthma.

Dosage: For children, a dose of 25 drops of standardized ivy leaf extract is recommended; for adults, 50–75 drops are used, depending on weight. The extract is usually taken in water, in a tea, or by itself. Germany's Commission E recommends 0.3 grams daily.

Side effects: Side effects include nausea and vomiting. Dermatitis has been reported following direct skin contact.

Precautions during pregnancy: Use in pregnancy is not recommended since the ingredient emetine can induce uterine contractions.

Drug interactions: No drug interactions have been reported with ivy leaf extract.

MARIJUANA

Type: Traditional Japanese (Kampo) herbal medicine

Uses: Appetite stimulant in AIDS and used to treat chemotherapy-related nausea

Active ingredients: Tetrahydrocannabinol (delta9-THC), cannabidiol (CBD), and cannabigerol (CBG)

Mechanism of action: Suspected bronchodilator

One of the most controversial botanicals for treating asthma is marijuana, an herb that is illegal in most states. Marijuana comes from the dried flowers of the hemp plant, *Cannabis sativa.* The primary active ingredients—tetrahydrocannabinol, cannabidiol, and cannabigerol—are undergoing active investigation for potential medicinal properties. Synthetic delta9-THC (dronabinol) is used to treat anxiety, glaucoma, nausea, pain, and lack of appetite. CBD and CBG may have anti-inflammatory and analgesic action—and this is where research is most promising.

While marijuana may have medicinal benefits, there are only a few studies that have examined marijuana in asthma. One study is a 1975 clinical trial with eight subjects who had "stable bronchial asthma." Following exposure to methacholine, these subjects were treated with 2 percent delta9-THC, which "produced a prompt correction of bronchospasm." The same researchers also treated exercise-induced asthma with THC and reported an "immediate reversal."[8] Another study examined the effects of THC aerosol on five asthmatics. Three reported symptom resolution, while the aerosol made symptoms worse in the other two.[9] Finally, a randomized, controlled trial involving ten asthmatics found that airway resistance decreased 10 to 13 percent in subjects who ingested 2 percent THC. These researchers also reported a modest reduction in airway resistance after subjects smoked marijuana.[10]

Perhaps the greatest hurdle marijuana must overcome for asthmatics is that most people smoke the herb. While marijuana may possess compounds that are active against asthma, marijuana combustion releases toxic compounds that can cause the lungs more harm than good.[11] Some people also have allergic and asthmatic reactions to *Cannabis.*[12] Add to this evidence that the smoked herb decreases exercise performance[13] and is a mind-altering agent, and you have a very mixed bag for marijuana.

Because marijuana continues to be a hot political and social issue, good research is hard to find. If marijuana has a future as an herbal remedy, it will be in the form of purified or synthesized compounds proven to be safe and efficacious. In the meantime, given the devastating quantity of free radicals delivered to the lungs from combustion, marijuana smoking is strongly discouraged. In fact, I consider marijuana smoke just as dangerous as tobacco smoke for asthmatics.

PETASITES HYBRIDUS (BLATTERDOCK, BOG RHUBARB, BOGSHORNS, BUTTERBUR, BUTTER-DOCK, BUTTERFLY DOCK, CAPDOCKIN, FLAPPERDOCK, LANGWORT, PESTWURZ, *PETASITES VULGARIS*, UMBRELLA LEAVES)

Uses: Asthma, cough, gastric ulcers, migraine, and overactive bladder

Active ingredients: The sesquiterpenes petasin and isopetasin, and flavonoids

Mechanisms of action: Anti-inflammatory and probable inhibition of leukotriene synthesis

Petasites hybridus is a perennial shrub found in Asia, Europe, and North America, which was used in the Middle Ages to treat the plague. Today, butterbur is used to treat migraine headaches, asthma, and bowel disorders. The leaves of this shrub can attain a diameter of three feet; allegedly the term "butterbur" originated from the leaves being used to wrap butter in the days before refrigeration.

Used by the Greeks to treat asthma, it is suspected that butterbur exerts its antiasthma effect by inhibiting leukotriene synthesis. Petasin, one of the active ingredients, is an antispasmodic that has anti-inflammatory action and inhibits leukotriene synthesis. The suspicion that butterbur has a positive effect on asthma is based on a study showing that *Petasites* extracts inhibited leukotriene production in the stomach.[14] There is only one trial on butterbur's impact on asthma, in which researchers examined the effect of *Petasites* rhizome powder (600 mg) on seventy individuals with asthma and bronchitis. According to the authors, a single dose of *Petasites* improved FEV_1.[15] While these results are encouraging, more studies are needed before we know whether *Petasites* has a significant role in asthma treatment.

Dosage: Most authorities recommend 50–100 mg of *Petasites* taken twice daily with meals. Standardized extracts usually contain at least 7.5 mg of petasin and isopetasin. Do not use any preparations that contain pyrrolizidine alkaloids.

Side effects: Liver toxicity is the most important side effect and is caused by pyrrolizidine alkaloids, which are normally removed from extracts. There are also reports of inhibited testosterone synthesis, but these findings have not been confirmed.

Precautions during pregnancy: Use in pregnancy and during lactation is inadvisable.

Drug interactions: No drug interactions with *Petasites hybridus* have been reported.

Special considerations: *Petasites hybridus* contains pyrrolizidine alkaloids that may be carcinogenic and can cause liver toxicity, so make sure to use a preparation without these alkaloids.

SAIBOKU–TO (CHAI-PU-TANG, TSUMURA SAIBOKU-TO, TJ-96)

Type: Traditional Japanese (Kampo) herbal medicine consisting of ten herbs—*Bupleuri radix, Glycyrrhiza glabra* (licorice, sweet root), hoelen, *Magnolia officinalis, Panax ginseng* (Asian ginseng, Chinese ginseng, Korean ginseng), *Perillae frutescens, Pinelliae tuber, Scutellaria baicalensis* (Chinese skullcap), *Zingiber officinale* (ginger), and *Zizyphus vulgaris*

Uses: Allergies and asthma

Active ingredients: Multiple active ingredients, including baicalein, davidigenin, dihydroxydihydromagnolol, flavonoids, glycyrrhizin, glycyrrhetinic acid, isoflavonoids, lignans, liquiritigenin, magnolol, medicarpin, oroxylin, saikosaponin, sterols, triterpenoids, saponins, wogonin, and phenolic compounds

Mechanisms of action: Apparent immunosuppressive and anti-inflamatory effects similar to steroids

Saiboku–to is a popular mixture of ten herbs used in China and Japan to treat asthma. Needless to say, when a mixture contains ten herbs, each with its own unique set of actions, the chemistry gets tricky. Despite these complexities, there is an impressive emerging body of literature regarding TJ-96. Researchers have picked this herbal potpourri apart and found that it inhibits leukotriene release and synthesis, steroid metabolism, eosinophil survival, histamine release, allergic reactions, and even possibly blood levels of IgE. This herbal mixture also allegedly helps steroid-dependent asthmatics reduce their steroid dose, a benefit known as "steroid sparing."

A study from the Saga Medical School in Japan, reported that Saiboku-to inhibited leukotriene B4 synthesis in animals.[16] Another study found that TJ-96 reduced bronchoconstriction in asthmatic guinea pigs.[17] (I didn't even know guinea pigs could get asthma!) One randomized study examined a three-month trial of Saiboku-to in 112 steroid-dependent asthmatics. Of those treated, 32.8 percent reported moderate improvement in symptoms and 60.9 percent reported slight improvement, compared to 10.4 percent and 29.1 percent, respectively, in the untreated group. This 1993 study did not, however, offer any objective evidence of enhanced lung function. The authors reported that, in the treatment group, 3.1 percent withdrew from steroid treatment completely and another 17 percent were able to reduce their steroid dose by over 50 percent.[18] Another study reported that three of nine asthmatics studied had a positive response to Saiboku-to,[19] and a Japanese study involving forty asthmatic patients recorded significant reductions in steroid use.[20]

More than a couple of favorable studies are needed to earn TJ-96 a place in the antiasthma argumentum. Nevertheless, given the popularity of Saiboku-to in Asia and some initially positive research, asthmatics searching for a botanical remedy may consider a trial of this herbal combination.

Dosage: The most common dosage used in Japan is 7.5 grams of powdered herb a day.

Selected side effects: The following is a list of side effects for some of the individual herbs in Saiboku-to:

Glycyrrhiza glabra—Possible side effects include hypertension, low blood potassium, elevated blood sodium, heart problems, testosterone synthesis inhibition, and water retention. Use of any product that contains more than one gram of glycyrrhizin is not recommended for more than two weeks. Glycyrrhizin-free licorice products are available and appear to have fewer side effects. Do not use licorice if you have kidney or liver problems.

Panax ginseng—Possible side effects include agitation, breast tenderness, insomnia, menstrual problems, and stomach upset. If you have high blood pressure, talk to your doctor before taking ginseng. Overdose can cause edema, insomnia, and hypertonia.

Scutellaria baicalensis—No significant side effects are reported.

Zingiber officinale—Possible side effects include heartburn. Talk to your doctor before taking *Zingiber* if you have a history of gallstones or are about to have surgery.

Precautions during pregnancy: Since *Glycyrrhiza glabra* and *Panax ginseng* are absolutely contraindicated during pregnancy, Saiboku-to use is also inadvisable.

Selected drug interactions: As is true in traditional pharmacology, the more agents you use, the greater the potential for interactions. The following is a list of drug interactions for some of the individual herbs in Saiboku-to:

Glycyrrhiza glabra—Interactions are reported with aspirin, corticosteroids (oral and topical), Coumadin, digitalis, digoxin, diuretics, etodolac, glycosides, ibuprofen, interferon, isoniazid, nabumetone, oxaprozin, risperidone, and warfarin. Licorice also increases diuretic-related potassium loss. If you are using any of these medications, check with your doctor before taking Saiboku-to.

Panax ginseng—Interactions are reported with alcohol, Coumadin, diabetes medications, flu vaccine, insulin, ticlopidine, Triotann-S Pediatric, and warfarin. If you are using any of these medications, check with your doctor before taking Saiboku-to.

Scutellaria baicalensis—No drug-herb interactions are reported.

Zingiber officinale—Interactions are reported with anesthetics, cancer chemotherapy, heparin, ticlopidine, and warfarin. If you are using any of these medications, check with your doctor before taking Saiboku-to.

Special considerations: People with gallbladder or gallstone problems should not take *Zingiber officinale* (ginger) without a doctor's permission. One study has also reported that Saiboku-to can interact with diazepam, so if you're taking this medication check with your physician before using Saiboku-to.

TYLOPHORA ASTHMATICA (*TYLOPHORA INDICA*, INDIAN IPECAC)

Type: Traditional Indian or Ayurvedic herbal medicine

Uses: Allergies, arthritis, asthma, bronchitis, and diarrhea

Active ingredients: Tylophorine and tylophorinine

Mechanisms of action: Anti-inflammatory and antihistamine

Native to eastern and southern India, *Tylophora* has been used in the treatment of allergies, arthritis, bronchitis, and diarrhea. The active ingredients are the alkaloids tylophorine and tylophorinine, which appear to have anti-inflammatory, antihistamine, and expectorant action. It is also suspected that these alkaloids stimulate the adrenal glands, causing them to increase natural steroid production.

Several studies have demonstrated that *Tylophora* can help people with asthma. One placebo-controlled, double-blind, crossover study found that one week of *Tylophora* leaf ingestion improved "maximum breathing capacity, vital capacity, and peak expiratory flow," with a reduced incidence of nocturnal asthma. This reduction in nocturnal asthma lasted up to twelve weeks.[21] Unfortunately, daytime asthma-related symptoms were not affected by *Tylophora.* Another double-blind, placebo-controlled study of 110 asthmatics, who each consumed one *Tylophora* leaf daily for six days, reported moderate to complete symptom relief in 62 percent of the *Tylophora* group, compared to 28 percent in the placebo group. Again, symptom relief persisted for up to twelve weeks.[22] A trial employing an alcohol extract of *Tylophora* reported similar results, with 58 percent of the treatment group experiencing improvement compared to 32 percent of the placebo group.[23]

Of all the herbal therapies reviewed, *Tylophora* is the one most extensively studied and documented for its ability to relieve asthma symptoms. While additional research is needed to clarify its role in asthma management, *Tylophora* is worthy of investigation by asthmatics seeking an herbal remedy.

Dosage: Typical dose is 200–400 mg of dried herb or 1–2 ml of tincture daily. Do not use *Tylophora* for more than two weeks.

Side effects: Side effects are usually seen with large doses and include stomach upset, oral pain, nausea, and vomiting. Nausea is a major drawback and is dose-dependent.

Precautions during pregnancy: Safety in pregnancy and lactation is unknown.

Drug interactions: No drug-herb interactions are reported.

chapter 9

Mind Over Asthma and Other Complementary Therapies

RELAXING IS HALF THE BATTLE in the war against asthma. Changing how you live is hard, but changing how you think is even harder. We cannot ignore the emotional impact of asthma or how emotions affect asthma.

Asthma and emotions often go hand in hand: how asthmatics feel has a lot to do with what goes on in their lungs. For many individuals, asthma is a complex interplay between mind and body, with attacks triggered by anger, stress, and even laughter. But there's nothing funny about asthma. Many people have irrational fears about asthma: they think asthma is the first step on a long and painful road to ill health or untimely death. Simply stated, for the overwhelming majority of asthmatics, these fears are unfounded. As we learned in Chapter 1, most asthmatics live healthy and active lives. Nevertheless, fear, anxiety, stress, and other negative emotions can trigger and exacerbate your asthma. By using the power of your mind to calm your emotions and alleviate stress, you can help free yourself from asthma.

EMOTIONS AND ASTHMA

Since the twelfth century, when Jewish philosopher and physician Maimonides (1135–1204) first observed the link between asthma and emotions, a tremendous body of literature has accumulated examining how negative emotions increase asthma risk. One study followed 5,231 adults for thirteen years and found that anxiety and depression were "independent predictors of asthma."[1] Negative emotions not only predispose people to asthma, they can make asthma worse. Multiple studies have documented that anxiety, depression, and inadequate social networks exacerbate asthma. Acute and chronic stress is particularly devastating; research demonstrates that some asthmatics feel worse when stressed.[2] In fact, emotions can radically alter lung function, and it is estimated that 20 to 45 percent of asthmatics experience bronchoconstriction when stressed.

Children are especially susceptible. Asthma is the fourth-leading cause of childhood disability, responsible for an estimated ten million lost school days. One study from the National Jewish Medical and Research Center in Colorado found that the "severity of asthma is related to increased emotional difficulties" in children.[3] Asthmatic children also tend to have more anxiety and medically related fears than non-asthmatic children.[4] University of Rochester School of Medicine scientists monitored lung function in twenty-four asthmatic children while they watched the movie *E.T. The Extra-Terrestrial.* The researchers found that emotions were "associated with increased airway reactivity and decreased pulmonary function," which persisted even after the movie ended.[5]

A study from North Dakota State University examined the relationship between lung function and social interactions in twenty asthmatics. While "mood and stressors" had the greatest impact on peak expiratory flow, social contacts had the most influence on symptoms; the authors concluding that "psychosocial variables were clearly related to [peak expiratory flow rate] and asthma symptoms."[6] Another study examined the effects of final examinations on a group of twenty mildly asthmatic college students and found that the number of eosinophils (which cause inflammation) increased significantly with stress. The authors concluded that the stress associated with final exams acts as a cofactor to increase airway inflammation and may enhance the severity of asthma.[7]

Not only can stress make the life of an asthmatic miserable, but there is also evidence that asthmatics are generally more depressed and anxious than the rest of the population. Poorly controlled asthmatics often experience depression and disruptions in their personal lives. One study of 230 asthmatics found that 45 percent were clinically depressed and that this depression directly influenced their symptoms.[8] Another study found that "anxiety and depression levels were noticeably higher in asthmatic patients than in patients with chronic liver disease and healthy subjects."[9] Does asthma cause depression or does depression cause asthma? It is reasonable to say that there is probably an element of truth to both of these assertions. Having asthma can certainly cause some people to become depressed and anxious, whereas depression and anxiety clearly appear to be risk factors for developing asthma. Regardless of what causes what, depression and anxiety take a devastating toll on asthmatics.

An even more dramatic reflection of this observation can be found in studies that examine asthma-related deaths. In a study on children who died from asthma, the authors concluded that these children had "exhibited emotional states of hopelessness and despair in the days immediately preceding their deaths."[10]

Researchers have also found a strong association between asthma and panic disorder, as well as "passive" or "repressive" coping styles. It is believed that panic leads to hyperventilation, which creates nervous system imbalances that predispose a person to asthma. These imbalances involve the autonomic nervous system, which is responsible for controlling bodily functions such as breathing and digestion. It is hypothesized that anxiety, panic, and passive-repressive coping result in a heightened autonomic sensitivity that leads to negative health consequences like bronchoconstriction. One study found that panic and repressive coping increase the risk of asthma morbidity.[11] This report suggests that panic sufferers benefit most from "relaxation-oriented methods," whereas asthmatics who cope through repression and/or panic benefit from therapies that increase their awareness of respiratory symptoms.

Social support and emotions can even influence how asthmatics respond to viral infections; one study found that "negative life events were associated with increased episodes of colds and asthma, but only when levels of social support were low."[12] Stress can also devastate immune function and increase the risk of infection in asthmatics. Multiple studies have documented the dramatic negative effects of acute and chronic stress on immune function, particularly impairing the effectiveness of natural killer cells and T lymphocytes. Finally, asthma symptoms are often worse at night, leading to sleep deprivation that results in an increased susceptibility to infection.

LEARNING TO RELAX

Almost every asthmatic knows from personal experience that anxiety, stress, and panic play important roles in asthma. Feeling their lungs tighten, many asthmatics become anxious and set in motion the vicious cycle of increasing anxiety and worsening symptoms. Throughout this book, I have asked you to carry out many difficult tasks—to exercise, eat right, and change your environment. I am now asking you to do the hardest thing of all: to change how you react emotionally to asthma. Every time you start to feel tightness in your chest, instead of thinking, "Oh no, I'm going to have an attack and die," start to think, "It's time to relax." Not an easy task, especially if you're used to years of panic.

Making the transformation from panic to calm can take months or years. How you make this transition is a matter of choice, as there are many paths to choose from. Known as complementary therapies, these paths encompass a wide range of non-pharmacological treatment options, from acupuncture to yoga. These therapies fall into three, often interrelated categories: breathing exercises, relaxation therapy, and analysis. Ideally, you can choose one that encompasses aspects of all three.

- Breathing therapies concentrate on breath control and are found in disciplines such as yoga and Buteyko breathing.
- Relaxation therapies include massage, chiropractic, biofeedback, and listening to music.
- Analysis involves thinking rationally about asthma and realizing that asthma can be controlled. While exercising, eating right, and making other lifestyle changes are critical to healing asthma, it's equally important to think about how emotions impact your life. You can ponder these thoughts while walking the beach or rock climbing, or with the aid of a therapist—it's up to you.

It's probably going to take some trial and error to find which techniques work best for you, but that's half the fun. Which technique you choose is not as important as making a choice, since choosing forces you to pay attention to the mind as well as the body. Paying attention to your feelings will not only help alleviate your asthma but also heal old wounds and rid your mind of negative emotional baggage. Each of us deserves to live a good life and be happy with who we are.

In this chapter, we'll review complementary therapies and present the latest scientific research supporting their use in asthma. There is an impressive body of literature on complementary treatments in asthma, the most effective therapies being those that emphasize proper breathing and long-term relaxation. Remember, however, that research on complementary therapies is subject to the same strengths and weaknesses found in all scientific endeavors.

My personal bias leans toward yoga coupled with some form of analysis. Yoga demands excellent breath control and is one of the best overall exercises. I also strongly suggest analysis, preferably with a psychologist or psychiatrist, as it is hard to imagine anyone walking away from asthma emotionally unscathed. A knowledgeable and caring professional can help you heal these wounds and grow as a person.

NEVER UNDERESTIMATE THE POWER OF SUGGESTION: THE PLACEBO EFFECT

Before we look at individual therapies, let's examine an area of potential confusion, a problem frequently encountered in research studies on complementary therapies: the "placebo effect." The placebo effect occurs when study subjects receive a placebo (an inert treatment or substance) and nonetheless report improvement because they *believe* the treatment is helping them. This is a common phenomenon in many placebo-controlled trials.

Scientists expect the placebo effect and use statistics to determine when outcome differences between treatment and placebo groups become important or "statistically significant." In other words, what researchers look for is an outcome difference between treatment and placebo groups that demonstrates that the treatment provides a measurable benefit beyond what would be expected from the placebo effect alone. By demonstrating this "statistically significant" difference, scientists can assert that the treatment actually works. Sometimes the outcome difference between placebo and treatment groups is so small as to be statistically insignificant; that is, the treatment offers no benefit beyond what would be expected from the placebo effect.

From personal experience, I have learned to respect the power of suggestion. Please don't tell anyone, but I have successfully used the power of positive thinking with many of my patients. Not surprisingly, there is a substantial body of literature affirming that the placebo effect is a potent part of many therapies and that believing something will work can actually influence the outcome. Perhaps one of the best examples of this mind/body phenomenon relates to the immune system: several studies have documented that suggestion under hypnosis can influence immune function in certain individuals.

Studies have also shown that a physician's attitude toward a particular therapy can influence the efficacy of that therapy. One study compared a group of patients who were offered a treatment by a physician who presented the information in a "positive manner" against another group who received the information in a "non-positive manner." The treatment itself was the same in both groups. After two weeks, there was a significant difference in patient satisfaction between the positive and negative groups, as "64 percent of those receiving a positive consultation got better, compared to 39 percent of those who received a negative consultation."[13]

The placebo effect represents the healing power of your mind and may be one of the reasons why the treatments discussed in this chapter can help people with asthma. What does this mean for you? While reading this book, if you discover that studies have not supported the use of your favorite therapy, do not stop using that therapy. The placebo effect may be playing a role in your particular case. Remember, what works for one person may not work for another. The only time you should abandon a therapy is if it may cause more harm than good. Bottom line: If the therapy works for you, use it.

ACUPUNCTURE

Acupuncture has been used in traditional Chinese medicine for over 3,000 years and employs needles strategically placed in "points" on the body. These needles balance the yin (passive) and yang (active) forces and attempt to restore health by increasing energy (known as *qi*) flow through the body's meridians or channels. Sometimes a small electric current is passed through the acupuncture needle to enhance this effect. There are about 365 specific acupuncture points— with several thousand additional points located bodywide—located mainly on the hands, head, and ears. While acupuncture is used in China to treat virtually any illness, in the West it is primarily employed in the treatment of chronic pain and substance abuse.

Studies have found that acupuncture can help people with asthma; however, results are mixed. One study from Denmark examined acupuncture versus placebo acupuncture in seventeen patients with stable bronchial asthma. The treatment group experienced an average 22 percent increase in morning peak flow, with a 53 percent reduction in beta-agonist use. These results differed significantly from the placebo group for the first two weeks of this study, but after two weeks similar results were observed. Of particular interest, the authors reported a significant decrease in IgE antibodies in the treatment group.[14] The Cochrane Database of Systematic Reviews, an evidence-based medical database, published an examination of seven studies involving 174 subjects, which concluded that "there is not enough evidence to make recommendations about the value of acupuncture in asthma treatment." The author continued to state that "further research needs to consider the complexities and different types of acupuncture."[15]

There remains a lack of consistent findings regarding acupuncture and asthma. While a strong recommendation cannot be made, if you have successfully used acupuncture, continue your treatments.

BIOFEEDBACK

Biofeedback trains people to influence bodily functions not normally under conscious control, such as breathing and blood pressure. Biofeedback uses machines to translate these biological functions into signals that the participant can recognize. For instance, in people who have had a stroke, a machine can recognize a muscle twitch in the affected limb and send a signal (such as a "beep") every time the muscle is twitched. By exerting conscious control over moving the limb with "feedback" from the beeps, the stroke victim may learn to use that limb again.

Biofeedback appears to be especially useful in medical conditions in which psychological factors play a significant role, such as chronic pain, anxiety, insomnia, and asthma. Biofeedback can help asthmatics with relaxation and breath control by training participants to take slow, deep diaphragmatic breaths to reduce anxiety.

Studies demonstrate that biofeedback reduces asthmatic symptoms, improves lung function, reduces medication use, and decreases emergency-room visits. In one study, participants reported decreased asthma severity, with a 50 percent reduction in bronchodilator use, following biofeedback training. Researchers also recorded an improved FEV_1/FVC ratio, an important objective measure of lung function. According to the authors, "significant differences were observed in the numbers of neutrophils and basophils in the trained group compared to controls, which supports the concept of decreased inflammation." These findings, though limited by the study size, suggest a positive role for biofeedback-assisted relaxation in non-steroid-dependent asthmatics.[16]

Another study from San Francisco State University used biofeedback with twenty-one asthmatics for fifteen months. Participants reported reduced asthma symptoms, medication use, emergency-room visits, and breathless episodes.[17] A similar study using relaxation biofeedback improved lung function by approximately 15 percent.[18] Finally, Ohio State University researchers reported that facial-relaxation biofeedback in children induced a more positive attitude toward asthma and lowered chronic anxiety. They did not, however, find any significant difference in self-rated asthma severity, medication use, or frequency of asthma attacks.[19]

There is also evidence that biofeedback can improve immune function. One study reported that, after eight sessions of biofeedback and relaxation therapy, subjects experienced significant increases in T-cell function, with decreased neutrophil and white blood cell counts—results that indicate reduced inflammation.[20]

Authorities suspect that decreased vagal tone and cholinergic activity are responsible for the observed effects of biofeedback on asthma. Vagal tone and cholinergic activity are part of the autonomic nervous system; decreased vagal tone may limit bronchial reactivity, and reduced cholinergic activity inhibits bronchoconstriction. There appears to be a downside, however, to reduced vagal tone in asthmatics. One study found that lung function actually decreased during therapy. While the decrease was short-lived, it did prompt researchers to conclude that it may be unwise for asthmatics to relax during an acute attack, because relaxation may produce a short-term decline in lung function and potentially exacerbate the asthma.[21]

While the ultimate role that biofeedback may play in asthma remains a topic of intense investigation, it is fair to say that biofeedback probably causes beneficial physiologic alterations that contribute to improvements in symptoms and lung function. Nonetheless, asthmatics should proceed with caution when using biofeedback, especially during an acute attack.

BUTEYKO BREATHING TECHNIQUE

For many asthmatics, the key to a better life may be learning how to breathe properly. Bad breathing has been variously called dysfunctional breathing, hyperventilation syndrome, and behavioral breathlessness. Whatever you call it, improper breathing can dramatically impact asthma. Multiple studies have documented the association between asthma and dysfunctional breathing, as well as the benefits of breathing therapy. In fact, hyperventilation is a leading suspect in exercise-induced asthma (EIA) and is probably the reason why asthma is more prevalent in athletes. Dysfunctional breathing is common in asthmatics: one survey found that 35 percent of female asthmatics and 20 percent of male asthmatics had dysfunctional breathing.[22] Considering how common breathing disorders are in asthmatics, it's safe to say that learning how to breathe correctly can go a long way toward improving the lives of many asthmatics.

Perhaps the best-known and most effective breathing therapy is Buteyko Breathing Technique (BBT). Buteyko Breathing corrects hyperventilation through diaphragmatic hypoventilation—instead of breathing too fast, BBT teaches asthmatics to breathe slowly, to "hypoventilate." Practitioners of BBT theorize that the method's effectiveness relies on elevated carbon dioxide (CO_2) levels in the blood; however, this is controversial. While we may not know exactly why BBT works, we do know that Buteyko Breathing does provide relief for many asthmatics.

One prospective, blinded, randomized Australian trial examined Buteyko Breathing in thirty-nine asthmatics who had substantial medication use. The Buteyko Breathing group had a "reduction in daily beta-agonist dose of 904 mcg, whereas the control group had a median reduction of 57 mcg." They also reported that daily steroid use fell 49 percent in the Buteyko group compared to no reduction in the control group.[23] Another study looked at thirty-six adults with mild to moderate asthma; after four weeks, those using BBT demonstrated a significant improvement in quality of life and reduced bronchodilator use.[24]

While additional studies are needed to confirm the efficacy of Buteyko Breathing for asthma, initial research is promising. Until then, the medical community remains hesitant to offer a definitive recommendation regarding BBT. However, breathing therapies have existed for centuries, and it is estimated that approximately 30 percent of asthmatics use some sort of breathing technique. The popularity of Buteyko Breathing speaks for itself, and I strongly recommend it as a viable complementary therapy. If you want to learn more about the Buteyko Breathing Technique, visit this website: www.wt.com.au/~pkolb/buteyko.htm.

CHIROPRACTIC

Chiropractic is based on the premise that the alignment of joints and muscles with each other and the spine influences health. Chiropractors treat disease by manual manipulation of these structures. While people who suffer from musculoskeletal pain often benefit from chiropractic manipulation, the impact of chiropractic on conditions like asthma is highly controversial. With respect to asthma, some chiropractors claim that manual manipulations reduce nervous system irritation, thereby relieving asthma symptoms.

Several studies have demonstrated that asthmatics feel better following chiropractic spinal manipulation. One study examined "active" versus placebo chiropractic spinal manipulation on thirty-six asthmatics undergoing standard medical therapy. The subjects received twenty treatments over a three-month period, after which the "active" group reported a 20 percent reduction in beta-agonist use, with a 10 to 28 percent improvement in quality-of-life scores. Researchers also found that asthma severity scores dropped 39 percent. Despite these promising results, the authors cautiously concluded that "the observed improvements are unlikely a result of the specific effects of chiropractic spinal manipulative therapy alone, but other aspects of the clinical encounter that should not be dismissed readily."[25]

A randomized, blinded, crossover study from Copenhagen compared one month of twice-weekly chiropractic spinal manipulation to placebo in thirty-one asthmatics who used bronchodilators and/or inhaled steroids. Though researchers did not report any change in objective lung function, they did find that airway hyperreactivity improved 36 percent and patient-rated asthma severity decreased 34 percent. While these results were encouraging, there were "no clinically important or statistically significant differences" between the active and placebo chiropractic interventions. The authors concluded that "the results do not support the hypothesis that chiropractic spinal manipulative therapy is superior to sham spinal manipulation in the management of pharmaceutically controlled chronic asthma in adults."[26] Nevertheless, the participants did subjectively feel better following therapy. Depending on your perspective, this can be just as important as finding objective clinical improvement.

So far, trials on chiropractic manipulation and asthma have failed to find any significant benefit despite reports of subjective improvement. A possible explanation for these findings can be found in studies that have observed that the simple act of touching can be therapeutic. This observation is especially true for therapies that involve a significant amount of manual manipulation.

The research on chiropractic and asthma offers an example of the placebo effect, with multiple studies demonstrating that the results of chiropractic manipulations equal those of placebo. Despite a lack of scientific validity, some asthmatics will benefit from chiropractic. This relief may occur because the act of being touched is relaxing, and relaxation can help people with asthma. Almost any therapy that results in stress reduction can potentially cause a subjective improvement in asthma symptoms. Not a surprising conclusion considering how emotions and anxiety often feed into the asthma equation.

As with other relaxation therapies, what works for one person may not work for another. If you feel better following chiropractic treatment, by all means continue visiting your chiropractor. Again, if it works, use it.

MUSIC THERAPY

Music therapy uses music to treat conditions like chronic pain. Despite famous asthmatic musicians like Beethoven and Leonard Bernstein, the scientific literature on music therapy and asthma is scant at best. One randomized, controlled study of music therapy involved seventy-two asthmatics who underwent eight music-therapy sessions. Lung function both improved and deteriorated during different treatment phases, but the authors concluded that "listening to music did not produce any specific therapeutic effects on asthma."[27]

There is, however, something to be said for playing a wind instrument. One study examined playing wind versus non-wind instruments in eighteen teenagers and found that the wind instrumentalists had a significantly more positive "asthma health" picture, perceiving themselves better able to cope with the disease.[28] Because serious vocalists and wind instrumentalists must develop precise breath control, it is suspected that this musical training, like breath training, can benefit asthmatics. According to experts, the pursed-lip expiratory breathing exercise common in breath training bears a remarkable resemblance to wind-instrument playing.[29] There are even anecdotal reports that asthma-related chest deformities (pectus carinatum and pectus excavatum) can be improved by playing a wind instrument. Whether or not you should buy a saxophone remains to be determined by additional studies.

YOGA

Yoga, a practice of mind/body unity, is built on the idea that easing the mind and reducing stress can improve your health. Though we do not understand the exact mechanisms behind the mind/body connection, yoga has proven beneficial for many asthmatics. Yoga works by combining breath control with meditative and therapeutic physical postures. Of all the complementary therapies, yoga is my personal favorite.

Multiple studies have established that yoga can reduce asthma symptoms, decrease medication use, improve exercise tolerance, and increase peak flow. One randomized, controlled study compared fifty-three asthmatics who performed an hour of yoga daily to a control group. The authors found that there was "a significantly greater improvement in the group who practiced yoga—in the weekly number of attacks of asthma, scores for drug treatment, and peak flow rate." Specifically, in the yoga group, the mean peak flow before yoga was 290.1 L/min compared to 362.8 L/min after yoga, a statistically significant difference.[30]

One study of forty-two moderate to severe asthmatics concluded that yoga therapy resulted in a significant increase in lung function and exercise tolerance, with fewer symptoms and reduced drug use.[31] In another trial, which examined Sahaja yoga in moderate to severe asthmatics using inhaled steroids, methacholine sensitivity declined and participants reported improved mood after four months of weekly yoga. The authors concluded that yoga had a beneficial effect on both objective and subjective measures of asthma.[32] Not surprisingly, these benefits disappeared after discontinuing yoga.

Yoga is one of the most extensively studied complementary therapies, and an impressive body of literature has accumulated supporting its use in asthma. From my own personal experience with yoga, I can say that this ancient art has helped me abort many asthma attacks simply by concentrating on how I breathe. Yoga directly influences the very essence of asthma—how we breathe—and is also a powerful form of exercise, emphasizing strength, flexibility, and balance.

PSYCHOTHERAPY

I believe that everyone with a medical condition should talk to someone about it—a psychiatrist, psychotherapist, church leader, your mother, or your spouse, anyone who will listen and who you trust. Consider talking with someone who gets paid to listen, such as a psychiatrist or psychologist, who can provide useful advice and insight. Unlike your mom or spouse, therapists are usually objective and have your interests in mind.

I strongly encourage psychotherapy, not only to help you deal with the emotions associated with having a chronic medical condition, but also because what goes on in the mind can have a definite impact on what happens in the lungs. This is especially true for children; multiple studies document that family-related stress has a devastating impact on childhood asthma. In fact, there is evidence that family therapy can dramatically improve asthma symptoms and lung function and is a useful adjunct to medication for asthmatic children.[33] Give analysis a try. If after a few sessions you are not getting results, you can start talking to your mom or spouse.

ASTHMA SUPPORT GROUPS

There is little doubt that being diagnosed with asthma is disturbing for many individuals. Fortunately, many communities sponsor support groups where people with asthma can develop friendships with others who understand their experiences and frustrations. Some people with potentially chronic medical conditions make the mistake of withdrawing from the world. This can truly be a tragic error, since humans by their very nature are social, and positive social interactions are necessary for survival. Having friends has profound health consequences, because positive social contacts protect against disease and death. In fact, asthmatics who are lonely or socially isolated often have poor outcomes and experience more severe symptoms.

If you want to learn more about asthma support groups in your area, check with the local office of the American Lung Association. The American Lung Association is also one of the best sources for general information and breaking news on asthma.

American Lung Association
1740 Broadway
New York, NY 10019
Phone: 212-315-8700 or 800-586-4872
Website: www.lungusa.org

If you're looking for an excuse to surf the web, there are several excellent on-line asthma support groups. They include:

- Sandwell Asthma Supporters Group (a support group based in England for people with asthma and emphysema): www.asthma-support.org.uk/wum.html
- Curing Asthma Support Group on Yahoo: www.egroups.com/group/asthmacured

Other excellent asthma-related websites include:

- About.com has a site containing useful information on how to start an asthma support group: www.asthma.about.com/library/weekly/aa050100a.htm
- Alt.Support.Asthma is packed with useful asthma information: www.radix.net/~mwg/asthma-gen.html

The University of California at Davis is home to the UC Davis Center for Complementary and Alternative Medical Research in Asthma. The Center was established in 1995 and is a leader in integrative and complementary asthma research.

Center for Complementary and Alternative
Medical Research in Asthma
University of California at Davis
One Shields Avenue, 3150B Meyer Hall
Davis, CA 95616-8669
Phone: 530-752-6575 • Fax: 530-752-1297

Website: www-camra.ucdavis.edu (ongoing research studies are available at www-camra.ucdavis.edu/currstudies.html)

OTHER HELPFUL THERAPIES

Multiple other therapies are available for asthma and could easily fill a book. Some of the therapies are elegant, and others are bizarre. What follows is only a small sample.

Perception Training

There is evidence that some asthmatics get into trouble because they have difficulty perceiving the start of an attack, thereby missing a chance to intervene early. Knowing this, researchers at the University of Ohio developed Perception Training, a program that helps asthmatics identify the early signs of an attack. Subjects were trained to recognize airway obstruction by breathing through a series of circuits that offered varying levels of resistance. Over time, the participants improved their ability to perceive airflow obstruction, potentially allowing them to begin therapy earlier.[34]

Nozovent

Simply stated, Nozovent keeps your nose open at night and increases nasal airflow. Our airways are designed to insure that the air we breathe contains the same amount of heat and moisture as the lungs. For asthmatics, nose breathing is preferable to mouth breathing as the nasal passages do a much better job of preheating and humidifying inhaled air. Authorities suspect that a major contributor to nocturnal asthma is nighttime mouth breathing caused by closed or clogged nasal passages. Swedish researchers tested this hypothesis by having fifteen patients with nocturnal asthma use Nozovent to reduce mouth breathing. Nozovent reduced asthma-related nighttime awakenings by almost 50 percent; twelve patients recorded fewer nocturnal symptoms, and seven patients used less nighttime medication.[35] Though additional studies are needed, given the noninvasive nature of this device, a trial of Nozovent is strongly recommended for people plagued by nocturnal asthma.

"DO SOMETHING ABOUT IT"

After reviewing the scientific literature, it becomes increasingly clear that relaxation therapies like massage or music therapy—therapies that require little or no active participation—offer limited benefits to people with asthma. In comparison, mind/body therapies like yoga or Buteyko Breathing—therapies that demand active participation—demonstrate, in study after study, the powerful role they can play in asthma management. These studies lend force to the saying "You can't get something for nothing." If you want to rid yourself of asthma, you have to work for it. While we can't expect a particular therapy to work for every asthmatic, yoga and breath training can improve the lives of many people with asthma.

The most important lesson is that people who relax and take control of their asthma end up with the best results. As is so often true, children—with their simple, no-nonsense approach—offer valuable lessons to adults. One study reviewed the coping techniques of children with asthma and found that two of the most effective strategies were, in the children's own words, "try to relax or stay calm" and "do something about it."[36] If adults took this attitude about all aspects of life, I suspect we'd all be better off. If you want to be free from asthma, you must take active control of your health.

chapter 10

Pharmacological Asthma Management

DESPITE OUR BEST EFFORTS, there will always be asthmatics who need medication to control their symptoms. Of all the asthma therapies discussed, it is the pharmacologic interventions that have consistently demonstrated the greatest efficacy. Without question, the best defense is a good offense: source control coupled with ventilation reign supreme when it comes to asthma. Drugs are certainly not the best way to treat any medical condition; however, for some asthmatics, medications will remain an occasional, and in some cases a permanent, fact of life.

There is no doubt that medications can cause problems of their own. While it is true that many medications have potentially disturbing and debilitating side effects, that some physicians rely too heavily on medications to treat asthma, and that many patients (including myself) have been overmedicated, it is also true that there are millions of people who might not be alive today had it not been for asthma medicine.

Yet again, knowledge is power. The more you know about the drugs you take, the more effective they will be. While the purpose of this book is to help you become medication-free or dramatically reduce the amount of medication you are taking, this chapter can help you avoid drug-related side effects while extracting the most benefit from pharmaceuticals.

ASTHMA DRUGS: AN OVERVIEW

Asthma drugs are roughly divided into two classes. The drugs in the first class promote smooth-muscle relaxation; they include beta2-adrenergic agonists, methylxanthines, and anticholinergics. These drugs are usually used for short-term control. Some medications like albuterol can be used to abort an acute asthma attack, known as "rescue" therapy. Bronchodilators that abort acute attacks treat asthma symptoms but not the underlying causes. Because these agents are intended for acute attacks, they often work in minutes and their effects usually last for only several hours.

The drugs in the second class prevent inflammation and include steroids, mast cell stabilizers, and leukotriene inhibitors. Unlike bronchodilators that act over a period of minutes to hours, anti-inflammatory drugs are usually intended for long-term control. Steroids and leukotriene inhibitors tend to be slow acting and are not normally used to abort an acute attack. These anti-inflammatory medications are used for long-term control in mild to severe asthmatics who have persistent symptoms. They are some of the most potent antiasthma agents available, with side effects that range from potentially highly toxic oral steroids to relatively safe leukotriene inhibitors.

ASTHMA SEVERITY CLASSIFICATIONS

Most physicians classify asthma severity into four categories: mild intermittent, mild persistent, moderate persistent, and severe persistent. With respect to asthma, the fundamental goal of all physicians is to minimize or totally abolish symptoms while preserving lung function with the least amount of medication. While the practice of medicine—being as much an art as a science—may vary among physicians, these general guidelines are used by most physicians when treating asthma. It should be understood, however, that no two asthmatics are exactly alike and your treatment plan needs to be individualized. Another important lesson is that while we grade asthma from mild to severe, even the mild asthmatic can have a severe attack under the right circumstances. While the following groupings are somewhat artificial, they do help doctors and patients think about asthma management.

Mild Intermittent Asthma

People with mild intermittent asthma usually have symptoms less than twice a week, with nighttime symptoms no more than twice monthly. These individuals feel well between attacks, which are short-lived and usually only last several hours to two days. FEV_1 stays above 80 percent of normal, and peak flow drops no more than 20 percent during an attack. Daily medication is not usually needed for mild intermittent asthma; a short-acting beta2-agonist is used for symptoms only as needed. Additional medication may be necessary for the occasional exacerbation brought on by a cold or other irritant. Most doctors will add an inhaled steroid if an individual with mild intermittent asthma is using a beta2-agonist more than twice a week.

Mild Persistent Asthma

Mild persistent asthmatics have symptoms more than twice a week, but no more than once a day. Nighttime symptoms can occur more than twice monthly, and symptoms potentially limit activity. FEV_1 remains over 80 percent of normal, with peak flow dropping no more than 30 percent during an attack. Individuals with mild persistent asthma are usually treated with low-dose inhaled steroids or a mast cell stabilizer. Short-acting beta2-agonists are also used as needed. Second-line therapy for mild persistent asthma includes theophylline. The leukotriene inhibitors are now considered a first-line therapy for mild persistent asthma and may ultimately replace inhaled steroids.

Moderate Persistent Asthma

Moderate persistent asthma is characterized by daily symptoms that have the potential to limit activity. During an attack, FEV_1 ranges from 60 to 80 percent of normal, with peak flow dropping more than 30 percent. Nocturnal symptoms can occur more than once weekly. Treatment can include a daily low to medium dose inhaled steroid coupled with a short- or long-acting beta2-agonist. Long-acting beta2-agonists are especially helpful in controlling nocturnal asthma. Theophylline is also occasionally used with leukotriene inhibitors, now considered a part of first-line therapy.

Severe Persistent Asthma

People with severe persistent asthma have severe daily and nighttime symptoms that significantly limit activity. FEV_1 is often less than 60 percent of normal, and peak flow routinely drops more than 30 percent during an attack. Individuals with severe persistent asthma need daily medications that may include short- or long-acting beta2-agonists coupled with a medium to high dose of inhaled or oral steroids. Theophylline is also used, as are leukotriene inhibitors.

ACTION PLANS: MANAGEMENT OF ACUTE ASTHMA ATTACKS

Your doctor should provide you with an "action plan" concerning what needs to be done during an acute attack. If you don't have an action plan, ask your doctor to give you one. While the majority of action plans include a short-acting beta2-agonist like albuterol, it is vital that your doctor provides you with an individualized plan. If your acute attack is caused by an environmental allergen, remove yourself or that allergen or irritant from the environment. If the attack does not resolve after following your action plan, call your doctor immediately or go to the nearest emergency room. Many people with asthma know when they are in trouble and need to seek help from the medical profession. Read Chapter 2 to learn more about how to gauge the severity of an asthma attack.

EXACERBATIONS, STEP DOWN, STEP UP, AND ROUTINE HEALTH MAINTENANCE

Standard medical guidelines require physicians to aggressively medicate poorly controlled asthmatics. In fact, it is not uncommon for even mild, normally stable asthmatics to be placed on a short course of oral steroids if their asthma gets out of control. This "step up" therapy may appear reckless; however, out-of-control asthma is dangerous and, for physicians, protecting life comes first. Hence, it is perfectly reasonable to hammer poorly controlled asthma into submission. If your asthma is out of control, don't be surprised if you end up heavily medicated. Expect to see your doctor weekly if not several times a week until your asthma is under control. Once your asthma is controlled, your physician will begin "step down" therapy by gradually reducing the dosage and number of medications you use. You'll ideally be on the lowest dose and the fewest number of medications necessary to keep your asthma stable.

Most physicians order lung-function tests at the first office visit, with repeat testing as needed. Depending on how well controlled your asthma is, most doctors will see you every one to six months. If your asthma is severe or difficult to control, you may be referred to an asthma specialist. You should also have an annual physical and flu shot. Influenza is a dangerous asthma trigger that no asthmatic can afford to get. Contrary to popular belief, the flu shot does not cause the flu nor will it absolutely prevent you from getting the flu. A flu shot can help you avoid the flu or reduce the severity of your symptoms should you get infected. Also, ask your doctor if a pneumonia vaccine is right for you.

ADRENERGIC AGONISTS

Adrenergic agonists are divided into three categories: catecholamines, resorcinols, and saligenins. The catecholamines, which are usually only given in the hospital, include epinephrine, isoproterenol, and isoetharine. Catecholamines have largely been replaced by resorcinols, such as fenoterol, metaproterenol, and terbutaline, typically inhaled agents with a duration of action of four to six hours.

Saligenins include inhaled agents like albuterol (salbutamol) and salmeterol. Albuterol is a short-acting beta2-agonist, and salmeterol is a long-acting beta2-agonist. They work by targeting beta2-receptors on airway smooth-muscle cells, causing them to relax. These agents also help remove irritants from the lungs and inhibit inflammatory mediator release. Inhalation is the preferred route for beta2-agonist administration, since inhalation permits direct lung interaction with the fewest side effects. Short-acting agents like albuterol are standard medical therapy for aborting an acute asthma attack. New long-acting beta2-agonists like salmeterol are only used for long-term control.

Metaproterenol (resorcinol)

Trade names: Alupent and Metaprel.

Side effects: Anxiety, cough, dizziness, headache, hypertension, irregular heart rhythm, muscle cramps, nausea, palpitations, shortness of breath, tremor, and vomiting.

Absolute contraindications: History of abnormally fast heart rate.

Drug interactions: Beta-blockers, diuretics, and tricyclic antidepressants.

Terbutaline (resorcinol)

Trade names: Brethaire, Brethine, and Bricanyl.

Side effects: Anxiety, angina, dizziness, headache, irregular heart rhythm, nausea, palpitations, and vomiting.

Drug interactions: Beta-blockers and diuretics.

Albuterol (saligenin)

Other name: Salbutamol.

Trade names: Novo-Salmol, Proventil, Ventolin, and Volmax.

Side effects: Agitation, angina, anxiety, cough, dizziness, flushing, hallucinations, headache, hypertension, irregular heart rhythms, low blood pressure, muscle cramps, nausea, palpitations, and vomiting.

How to Use a Beta-Agonist Inhaler (Metered Dose Inhaler)

I am constantly amazed by how some people incorrectly use inhalers and by how some doctors instruct their patients in inhaler use. So, here are some easy instructions.

A typical inhaler includes a canister, an actuator, and a cap that covers the mouthpiece. The canister is a metal container that holds the medication, and the actuator is the plastic device that holds the canister and directs the medication into the mouthpiece. The mouthpiece, as the name implies, is the part of the actuator that goes into your mouth. You can tell which end of the actuator is the mouthpiece by the presence of a cap that covers the mouthpiece. The cap is intended to keep the actuator dirt-free. Officially, you should recap the actuator after each use; however, if you're like me, the cap may get trashed with the instructions (but try to not let that happen).

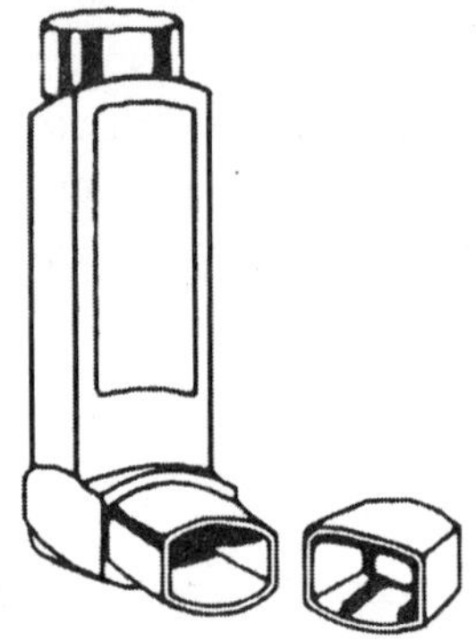

Figure 10.1. Typical inhaler.

Shake the inhaler five to ten times, then remove the cap. (We do not want you to inhale the cap.) Inspect the inside of the inhaler for any foreign objects and remove them. Make sure the medication canister is securely inserted in the actuator.

Brace the inhaler with your middle finger while wedging it between your thumb and index finger. Your thumb should be placed on the bottom of the inhaler while your index finger rests on top of the canister. Exhale as much air from your lungs as possible. Once you have emptied your lungs, place the mouthpiece one to two inches away from your mouth while keeping the actuator in an upright position. You'd be amazed by the contortions some people go through when using inhalers—upside down, sideways, you name it, any way but up. Ask your physician where you should position the inhaler in relation to your mouth; some inhalers need to be kept in front of the mouth, others are intended to be placed in the mouth, and some should be used with a spacer.

Using your index finger, depress the medication canister while taking a slow, deep breath through your mouth. This slow and deep breath should begin just as you depress the canister and will ideally last three to five seconds. You should feel a slight pressure as the medication enters your mouth. If you have trouble aiming the inhaler toward your mouth, you can cheat by wrapping your lips firmly about the mouthpiece and then depressing the canister while taking a slow and deep breath. If you have a new inhaler or have not used your inhaler for a month or more, make sure it's working by performing four "test sprays" away from your face and into the air before using.

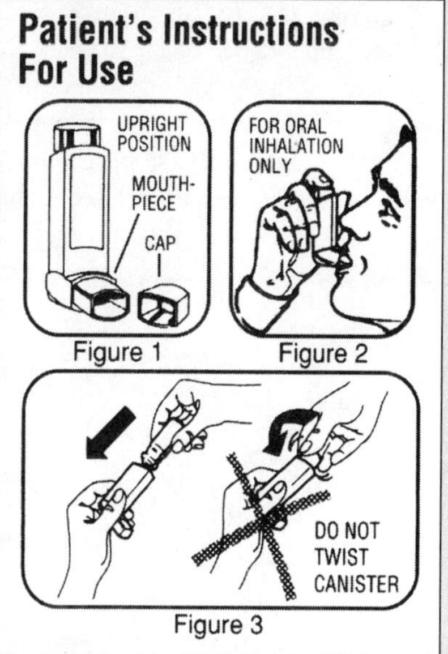

Figure 10.2. Proper inhaler holding and depressing technique.

After inhaling, hold your breath for ten seconds. While holding your breath, move the inhaler away from your face and take your finger off the canister. After ten seconds, exhale, wait one minute, then repeat the procedure. Most people use two inhalations; however, your doctor may instruct you to use a different amount. Waiting a minute between inhalations is necessary for short-acting beta2-agonists but not for most other inhaled medications, so be sure to ask your doctor how long you should wait between inhalations. These procedures also apply to inhaled steroids, except that the interval between inhalations is approximately thirty seconds. Always remember to rinse your mouth thoroughly after using an inhaled steroid to prevent thrush (a yeast infection of the mouth) and systemic absorption.

Some adults, but especially children, have trouble correctly aiming inhalers, with the medication landing on the tongue or throat. For this reason, "spacers" are available that hold the aerosolized medicine and permit a more uniform medication delivery. Spacers are also recommended for people who use inhaled steroids, to help prevent thrush.

Using a spacer is easy. All you need to do is attach the spacer to the actuator mouthpiece. Shake the actuator five to ten times, exhale, place the mouthpiece into your mouth, depress the canister to deliver a dose of medication into the spacer, then inhale. Remove the spacer mouthpiece from your mouth and hold your breath for ten to fifteen seconds, then exhale. Wait the prescribed time and repeat as directed by your doctor. Some spacers come with a face mask that is especially helpful for children.

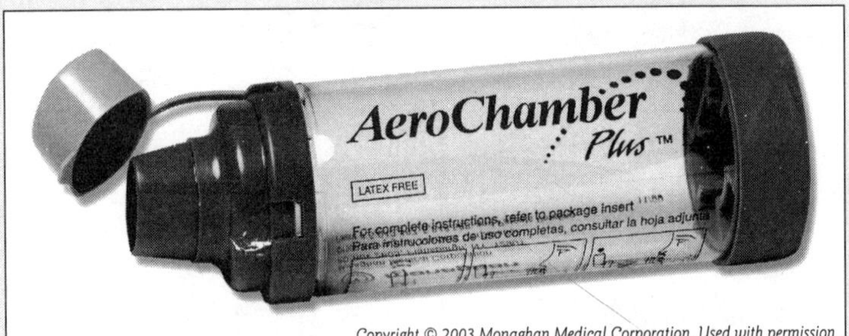

Copyright © 2003 Monaghan Medical Corporation. Used with permission.

Figure 10.3. AeroChamber Plus spacer (above) and basic technique (below).

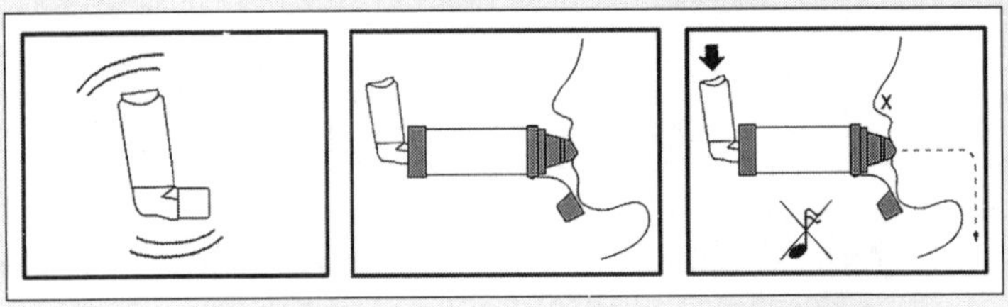

After using the inhaler, remove the metal canister from the actuator and wash the plastic actuator, mouthpiece, and cap with warm water. Shake off excess water and allow the actuator and mouthpiece cap to air-dry completely. Once dry, reinsert the medication canister into the actuator. Place the mouthpiece cap on the actuator mouthpiece. You should clean your inhaler daily.

To check how much medicine is left in an inhaler, some authorities suggest placing the canister in a pot of water to observe how it floats. While this technique allows a rough estimation of the remaining medication, it is not always accurate. I suggest you ask your doctor or pharmacist how many inhalations your canister contains and simply keep count. You can also purchase a DoseMonitor, which keeps track of the number of doses delivered and the time since the last dose.

Absolute contraindications: History of abnormally fast heart rate or severe heart disease.

Drug interactions: Beta-blockers, diuretics, and tricyclic antidepressants.

Salmeterol (saligenin)

Trade name: Serevent.

Side effects: Agitation, anxiety, bronchospasm, cough, dizziness, headache, hypertension, irregular heart rhythms, muscle cramps, nausea, palpitations, shortness of breath, and vomiting.

Absolute contraindications: Acute asthma attack or worsening asthma.

Special considerations: Salmeterol is a long-acting beta2-agonist, so giving extra doses is not recommended and can cause additive side effects. Discontinue use and call your physician if you experience chest pain, dizziness, headache, palpitations, tremors, or an irregular or rapid heart rate.

METHYLXANTHINES (THEOPHYLLINE)

Methylxanthines increase levels of cAMP (cyclic adenosine monophosphate), a cellular messenger that is involved in airway tone and causes bronchodilation. Several methylxanthines exist; however, theophylline is the most popular. It is considered a medium-potency bronchodilator, intended for long-term asthma control. Theophylline is not indicated for the treatment of an acute attack.

Theophylline

Trade names: Asmalix, Elixophyllin, Quibron-T, Quibron–T/SR, Respbid, Slo-Bid Gyrocaps, Slo-Phyllin, Theo-24, Theochron, Theobid Duracaps, Theo-Dur, Theo-Dur Sprinkle, Theolair, Theolair-SR, Theospan SR, Theo-Time, Theo-X, T-Phyl, Truxophylline, Uni-Dur, and Uniphyl.

Side effects: The most common side effects are agitation, anorexia, anxiety, diarrhea, dizziness, flushing, headache, insomnia, itching, nausea, nervousness, reflux, stomach pain, urinary frequency, and vomiting. More serious and potentially deadly side effects include seizures and abnormal heart rhythm.

Absolute contraindications: History of a fast, abnormal heart rate, peptic ulcer disease, or a history of seizures.

Nebulizers

Despite their best efforts, some people just don't have a happy relationship with their inhaler and end up depositing the medication on their tongue, dining-room set, or their neighbor's backyard. If you're one of these people, don't despair—switch to a nebulizer. A nebulizer uses compressed air and sterile saline to convert asthma medication into a fine, easy-to-inhale mist. People who benefit most from nebulizers are children, severe asthmatics, and individuals who are tired of medicating everything but their lungs.

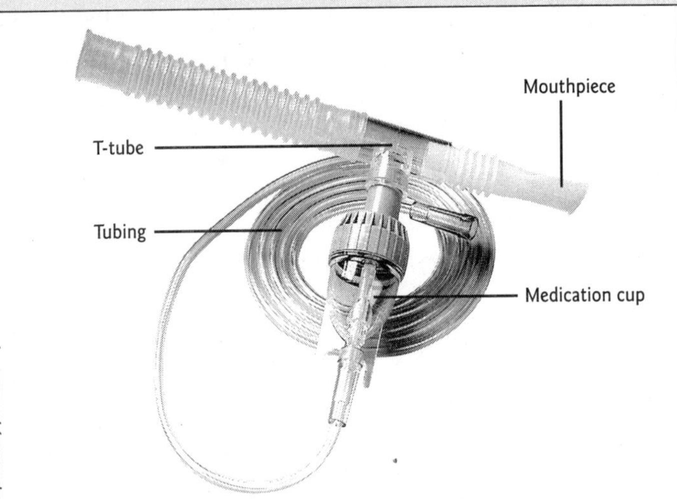

Figure 10.4. Typical nebulizer showing mouthpiece, medication cup, T-tube, and tubing.

The typical nebulizer has four parts: mouthpiece, T-tube, medication cup, and tubing that attaches to a compressor. Nebulizers can be used with a mouthpiece or a face mask. A mouthpiece is preferred since it delivers more medicine; however, a face mask is recommended for children under the age of two. Most people use premixed medication or saline preparations; some individuals use an eyedropper or syringe to draw up the medication that is then mixed with sterile saline. Your doctor will advise you on which method to use.

To use a nebulizer, place the prescribed amount of medication and saline in the medication cup. Attach the mouthpiece and then the medication cup to the T-tube. For children under the age of two, attach the face mask to the T-tube. Seal your lips firmly around the mouthpiece or place the mask on the child's face, then turn on the air compressor. Most machines require that you attach the tubing to the compressor outlet port prior to starting the nebulizer. Breathe slowly and deeply through your mouth, holding each breath for two to three seconds before exhaling. Continue this slow, deep breathing until all the medicine is used from the medication cup; most treatments last about ten minutes. Repeat this process as directed by your physician.

It is vital to follow the manufacturer's directions with regard to routine nebulizer maintenance and cleaning. Cleaning your nebulizer regularly is critical in order to maintain excellent working order and prevent medication build up. Most important, regular cleaning keeps the nebulizer germ-free, as dangerous lung infections can result from improperly maintained machines. After each use, clean the mouthpiece, medication cup, syringe or eyedropper, and T-tube with warm, distilled or sterile water for at least thirty seconds. After shaking off the excess water, allow these parts to air-dry on a clean towel, preferably overnight. Never clean the tubing. Once dried, reconnect the mouthpiece, T-tube, and cup to the air compressor and turn the machine on for thirty seconds to complete the drying process. Once this is done, disconnect the tubing, mouthpiece, T-tube, and cup, and store in a clean, dry area, preferably in a plastic bag. Clean the air compressor with an alcohol wipe once weekly. Since water and electricity don't mix, never put your air compressor in water.

Drug interactions: Adenosine, allopurinol, aminoglutethimide, amiodarone, barbiturates, carbamazepine, cimetidine, ciprofloxacin, disulfiram, enoxacin, erythromycin, fluvoxamine, imipenem, interferon alpha, isoniazid, lithium, metoprolol, mexiletine, moricizine, norfloxacin, pefloxacin, pentoxifylline, phenytoin, propafenone, propranolol, radioactive iodine, rifampin, ritonavir, Synthroid, thyroxin, tacrine, thiabendazole, ticlopidine, troleandomycin, and verapamil.

Special considerations: Theophylline blood levels must be checked for toxicity. The ideal theophylline level is 10–20 mcg/ml; however, some authorities recommend 5–15 mcg/ml. Call your doctor if you develop a fever while taking theophylline, since fever increases toxicity risk. Also, avoid tobacco, as it interferes with theophylline.

ANTICHOLINERGICS (IPRATROPIUM BROMIDE)

Anticholinergics promote bronchodilation, but are rarely used as first-line therapy because of their high side-effect profile. Like methylxanthines, while there are many anticholinergic drugs on the market, ipratropium bromide is the one most commonly used in treating asthma. Ipratropium has earned a niche by exhibiting a low side-effect profile and demonstrating itself as relatively safe for asthmatics with heart disease. The major drawback to this newer anticholinergic is that it is not a potent bronchodilator and has a slow onset of action; hence, it is not considered first-line therapy.

Ipratropium Bromide

Trade name: Atrovent.

Side effects: Abdominal cramps, agitation, anxiety, blurred vision, cough, dizziness, dry mouth, headache, nausea, palpitations, and vomiting. Atrovent can occasionally cause bronchospasm.

Drug interactions: No drug interactions have been reported.

STEROIDS

Steroids (corticosteroids, glucocorticoids) are the most powerful asthma medications for reducing inflammation. This power, however, comes with a price: all steroids, but especially oral steroids, have the potential to demonstrate significant toxicity and side effects. Contrary to popular belief, steroids are not true bronchodilators and this is why they are not usually used to abort an acute attack.

Inhaled Steroids

Inhaled steroids are first-line therapy for persistent mild to severe asthma. Intended for long-term control, inhaled steroids are usually used by asthmatics whose symptoms would otherwise require frequent beta2-agonist use. They are not normally prescribed for individuals with EIA or symptoms that are brought on by specific and avoidable triggers. Inhaled steroids have revolutionized asthma management by helping many asthmatics avoid oral steroids.

Dosing is variable, but the usual maintenance dose is two to four inhalations a day. Since inhaled steroids can take over a week to work, they are not effective in aborting acute attacks. While boasting a low side-effect profile, these agents, like oral steroids, can still produce devastating side effects. This is especially true when dosages exceed 400 mcg a day in children or 800 mcg a day in adults over prolonged periods of time. With typical use, however, the most common side effects are thrush and hoarseness. People who are at increased risk for more serious side effects include children (who can experience growth retardation), postmenopausal women, and individuals with inadequate dietary vitamin D and calcium. Several simple steps can help prevent complications from inhaled steroids:

1. Use the lowest dose of inhaled steroid possible.
2. Use a large volume-spacer device.
3. Rinse your mouth out with water after each dose of inhaled steroid.
4. Take dietary supplements: 800 mg of calcium and 250–500 IU of vitamin D, daily.

Beclomethasone

Trade names: Beclodisk, Becloforte, Beconase, Vancenase, and Vanceril.

Side effects: Adrenal suppression, dry mouth, earache, headache, itch, mouth or nose irritation, nasal ulcer/perforation, sneezing, and thrush.

Absolute contraindications: Active lung, mouth, or throat infection.

Drug interactions: No drug interactions have been reported.

Budesonide

Trade names: Pulmicort Turbuhaler and Rhinocort.

Side effects: Cough, dry mouth, nosebleed, throat pain, and thrush.

Drug interactions: No drug interactions have been reported.

Flunisolide

Trade Names: AeroBid, Bronalide, Nasalide, Nasarel, and Rhinalar.

Side effects: Agitation, dizziness, dry mouth, hoarse voice, itching, nasal congestion, nervousness, nosebleed or pain, sneezing, throat pain, and thrush.

Absolute contraindications: Active nasal infection.

Drug interactions: No drug interactions have been reported.

Fluticasone

Trade names: Flonase and Flovent.

Side effects: Facial swelling (angioedema), headache, itch, muscle pain, nasal congestion, sinus infection, and thrush. Fluticasone can rarely cause bronchospasm.

Absolute contraindications: Active infection and tuberculosis.

Drug interactions: No drug interactions have been reported.

Oral and Intravenous Steroids

The medications of last resort, oral steroids are usually only used in moderate to severe asthma when chronic disease fails to respond or worsens after conventional aggressive therapy. Oral or intravenous steroids are also occasionally used in mild to severe asthmatics who experience an acute attack that does not respond to aggressive bronchodilator therapy. We also sometimes see oral steroids like prednisone given to asthmatics who have short-term exacerbations, as from a cold. Oral steroids are not first-line therapy for an acute attack since their onset of action can take up to six hours.

While the optimal dose of oral steroid must be individualized, an initial starting dose of 20–60 mg a day is common. The goal of therapy is to use the absolute minimum dose. For steroid-dependent asthmatics, "alternate day therapy" is preferred—that is, taking steroids only every other day. Alternative day steroid therapy has fewer side effects, which is especially important for children, in whom growth retardation can result from steroid use.

"Tapering" is when a doctor slowly decreases the steroid dose, usually reducing the daily dose 5–10 mg every third or fourth day until the desired dosage is achieved. More rapid steroid tapers are occasionally employed, but this decision should be made by your physician. Tapering steroids slowly is critical because asthma symptoms tend to return when steroids are tapered too quickly. Also, corticosteroids suppress the adrenal glands, and we need to give these glands time to resume normal function before stopping steroid use completely. Suppression of the pituitary-adrenal axis is the most profound and dangerous side effect of steroid use; it is the chief cause behind many steroid-related side effects. The pituitary-adrenal axis is responsible for making vital hormones that regulate basic bodily functions like blood pressure. People who taper steroids too rapidly, or stop taking their steroids abruptly, can experience potentially dangerous and deadly low blood pressure. Therefore, it is critical to work with your physician closely when tapering steroids.

Prednisone

Trade names: Deltasone, Liquid Pred, Meticorten, Orasone, Panasol-S, Prednicen-M, Sterapred, and Winpred.

Side effects: See the next section, entitled "Steroid Survival Guide," for a discussion of side effects.

Absolute contraindications: Active fungal infection.

Drug interactions: Interactions have been reported with aminoglutethimide, aspirin, barbiturates, carbamazepine, cholestyramine, clarithromycin, colestipol, cyclosporine, diabetes medications, erythromycin, estrogen, isoniazid, ketoconazole, rifampin, salicylates, and troleandomycin.

Special considerations: Do not stop or taper steroids without a doctor's permission. Make sure you have a bone mineral density test and an annual eye examination to detect potential complications early. Consider wearing a medical alert bracelet or tag if you are chronically taking steroids. Continue seeing your physician as directed.

MAST CELL STABILIZERS

As we learned in Chapter 2, histamine is one of many asthma chemical mediators that reside in mast cells. Stabilizers like cromolyn sodium and nedocromil prevent mast cells from releasing chemical mediators and are especially helpful in allergic asthma, where histamine plays a critical role. Since mast cell stabilizers can take six weeks to work, they are intended for long-term control and are not useful during an acute attack. They can, however, prevent an attack if given prophylactically, before exposure to a known trigger such as exercise or cold air. For instance, cromolyn sodium can prevent EIA if given one hour before exercise.

Cromolyn Sodium

Trade names: Intal, Nalcrom, and Nasalcrom.

Side effects: Dizziness, cough, headache, hoarse voice, nasal congestion or pain, and throat pain.

Drug interactions: No drug interactions have been reported.

LEUKOTRIENE INHIBITORS

Leukotriene inhibitors have emerged as one of the most powerful antiasthma medications. Two basic mechanisms underlie the action of leukotriene inhibitors: Inhibitors like zileuton interfere with 5-lipooxygenase, the enzyme responsible for leukotriene synthesis. Zafirlukast and montelukast work by antagonizing the leukotriene receptor LTD4, thereby preventing the transmission of the chemical messages responsible for the asthma cascade.

Steroid Survival Guide

Steroids are an unfortunate fact of life for some people with asthma, inflammatory bowel disease, autoimmune disease, and rheumatoid arthritis. The good news for asthmatics is that if they follow the advice given in this book, they will probably be able to stop—or at the very least, dramatically reduce—steroid use. If you are a steroid-dependent asthmatic or feel that you are heading in that direction, talk to your doctor about taking a "steroid-sparing" agent like methotrexate. Studies have shown that steroid-sparing agents can help asthmatics reduce their steroid use by up to 50 percent.

Steroids are the medication of last resort for asthmatics, because of their high and often irreversible side effects. Unfortunately for steroid users, many of these side effects cannot be prevented. What follows is a list of potential side effects and how to avoid some of them.

- **Adrenal suppression**—There is no way to avoid adrenal suppression when taking oral steroids. The adrenal glands rest on top of your kidneys and normally produce steroid hormones. When this job is taken over by oral steroids, the adrenal glands markedly curtail steroid synthesis. Steroids are tapered gradually, and never discontinued abruptly, so that the adrenal glands can start making natural steroids again. The best way to prevent adrenal suppression is to use as little steroid as possible. If you must use steroids, ask your physician about "alternate day therapy," which can limit adrenal suppression and help avoid steroid-induced side effects.

- **Avascular necrosis**—A potentially debilitating complication, avascular necrosis occurs when a bone's blood supply becomes inadequate, resulting in bone death. Avascular necrosis usually involves the hip or shoulder. Treatment ranges from physical therapy to joint replacement.

- **Cataracts**—Cataracts are another complication of prolonged steroid use, so have your eyes checked annually by an ophthalmologist. Fortunately, cataracts are treatable.

- **Diabetes**—Steroids elevate blood sugar and can be especially dangerous for diabetics. The best defense against steroid-induced diabetes is to adopt a healthy diet and an exercise routine. Also, have your blood sugar checked regularly. It is usually not necessary for nondiabetic steroid users to take diabetes medications. There is emerging evidence that 600 mcg of chromium picolinate a day can help prevent steroid-related diabetes.

- **Fat redistribution**—Perhaps one of the most psychologically disturbing side effects of steroid use is the redistribution of fat to the face, neck, and abdomen—the so-called Cushingoid habitus. Some steroid-dependent asthmatics even develop a "buffalo hump" on their back, the result of fat deposition to the upper back. While fat redistribution cannot be prevented, a healthy diet coupled with regular aerobic and anaerobic exercise will help prevent steroid-associated weight gain.
- **Glaucoma**—Like cataracts, the best way to avoid steroid-induced glaucoma is to use as little steroid as possible. Steroid users should be tested for glaucoma annually.
- **Growth retardation**—This is primarily a problem for children. With the exception of eliminating steroid use, there is no way to prevent growth retardation in children who are steroid dependent. A child or adolescent who uses steroids needs to be examined regularly by a pediatrician.
- **High blood pressure**—Steroids cause sodium and water retention, thereby increasing blood pressure. While you can't prevent steroid-induced water retention, you can control your blood pressure by eating a healthy, low-salt diet and engaging in regular aerobic exercise.
- **Immune suppression**—While immune suppression may be desirable in illnesses like inflammatory bowel disease, immune suppression in an asthmatic can spell disaster by hampering the body's ability to fight infections. The best way to keep your immune system strong is to eat a healthy diet while getting enough sleep and exercise. Also, wash your hands regularly to prevent viral infections, and try to avoid people who are sick with the flu or common cold. Consider supplementing your diet with daily vitamin C (1,000 mg), vitamin E (200 IU), and zinc (25 mg) to boost immune function.
- **Impaired wound healing**—Impaired wound healing is a problem for many steroid users. Apply antibiotic ointment to cuts and abrasions, then cover the wound with a dry, sterile bandage. Call your doctor if you see pus draining from a wound or if the wound appears infected. Finally, consider taking zinc (220 mg) and vitamin C (1,000 mg) daily to aid wound healing.
- **Myopathy**—Steroids can weaken your muscles; however, regular weight training will keep your muscles fit.

- **Osteoporosis**—Perhaps the most feared steroid-induced complication is osteoporosis, a weakening of the bones that can lead to bone fractures, especially of the hip. According to the American College of Rheumatology (ACR), anyone who takes oral steroids for over six months should have a spine and/or hip bone mineral density examination at the beginning of therapy and every six to twelve months thereafter. The ACR also recommends daily calcium (800 mg) and vitamin D (250–500 IU) for people who use an average of 15 mg of steroid daily. An alternative regimen is daily calcium with alfacalcidol (1 mcg) or calcitriol (0.5 mcg), active forms of vitamin D. Talk to your doctor about which regimen is best for you. If you decide to take activated vitamin D, make sure your doctor checks you for elevated blood levels of calcium and uric acid, side effects that can occur during therapy. From my perspective, the ACR recommendations are low, so I recommend 1,000 mg of calcium with 400–800 IU of vitamin D daily.

  Men should have their testosterone levels checked. According to the American Association of Clinical Endocrinologists and the American College of Endocrinology, men with low testosterone should have replacement therapy. Authorities also recommend bone-building bisphosphonates, such as alendronate or risedronate, for the prevention and treatment of steroid-induced osteoporosis. Talk to your physician about new agents like alfacalcidol that are being developed to help prevent steroid-induced osteoporosis. Smoking cessation, reducing or eliminating alcohol, and beginning a program of weight-bearing exercise can help prevent steroid-induced osteoporosis.

- **Pancreatitis**—Inflammation of the pancreas, a painful complication of steroid use, is mercifully rare; however, if you experience a sudden onset of stomach pain while taking steroids, call your doctor right away or go to the nearest emergency room.

- **Peptic ulcer disease**—Steroids are brutal on the stomach and can cause irritation and ulcers. Avoiding tobacco, alcohol, aspirin, and NSAIDs helps prevent steroid-induced stomach disease. Some doctors prescribe proton-pump inhibitors to protect the stomach during steroid therapy.

- **Pseudotumor cerebri**—This is a rare complication characterized by increased intracranial pressure that causes a persistent, potentially severe headache. Call your doctor if you have a headache that does not go away.

- **Psychological problems**—Steroids can cause psychological problems, ranging from irritability to psychosis. These side effects are uncommon; however, if you see or hear things you know are not real, call your doctor immediately or go to an emergency room.
- **Striae**—Striae are stretch marks caused by rapid weight gain that are most commonly found on the abdomen, underarms, and thighs. The best way to prevent striae is to control your weight through diet and regular exercise.
- **Thin skin**—Thin skin is a complication of long-term steroid use that can only be avoided by not taking steroids.
- **Vitamin and mineral interactions**—Since steroids can cause magnesium deficiency, daily magnesium (300–400 mg) is recommended for individuals who use steroids for two weeks or more. Similar recommendations apply to vitamin B_6, with 2 mg daily being the standard dose. Steroids can also cause potassium wasting, which can be offset by increased intake of fruits and vegetables, especially bananas.
- **Weight gain**—For many steroid users, weight gain is the most troubling complication. Fortunately, obesity can be prevented by adhering to a healthy diet together with a program of aerobic and anaerobic exercise.

Leukotriene inhibitors can dramatically reduce symptoms and have allowed many asthmatics to discontinue or significantly reduce steroid use. While effectively preventing exercise-induced and nocturnal asthma, leukotriene inhibitors are not indicated for allergic asthma. In fact, it is estimated that less than 50 percent of asthmatics derive benefit from these agents. Given this consideration, most physicians discontinue their use if there is no improvement in symptoms after four weeks of therapy.

Zileuton

Trade name: Zyflo.

Side effects: Dizziness, fatigue, headache, insomnia, itch, nausea, stomach pain, and rash.

Absolute contraindications: Liver disease.

Drug interactions: No drug interactions have been reported.

Special considerations: Monitor with blood tests, as ordered by your physician.

Zafirlukast

Trade name: Accolate.

Side effects: Cough, dry mouth, fatigue, headache, runny nose, sore throat, and stomach pain. Zafirlukast can rarely cause bronchospasm.

Drug interactions: Astemizole, terfenadine, and warfarin.

Special considerations: Liver function tests may be needed, as ordered by your physician.

Montelukast

Trade name: Singulair.

Side effects: Headache, fatigue, fever, and stomach pain.

Drug interactions: Phenobarbital and rifampin.

EXPECTORANTS AND MUCOLYTIC AGENTS

Though expectorants may help with airway secretions, they have no established role in the treatment of asthma and little impact on bronchoconstriction or inflammation. The same can be said of mucus-loosening agents like acetylcysteine, which may actually cause bronchoconstriction in sensitive individuals.

MEDICATIONS TO AVOID: BETA-BLOCKERS, ASPIRIN, AND NSAIDS

Beta-blockers, used for hypertension, heart disease, and glaucoma, should be absolutely avoided by people with asthma. Beta-blocker medications include Apo-Nadol, atenolol, Betaloc, Betimol, Blocadren, Corgard, Inderal, Lopresor, Lopressor, metoprolol, nadolol, Novo-Nadolol, Nu-Metop, propranolol, Syn-Nadolol, Tenoretic, Tenormin, Timolide, timolol, Timoptic, and Toprol XL. If you are using a beta-blocker, don't stop taking the medication; rather, call your doctor for further instructions. While beta-blockers in asthma are usually contraindicated, there are some special circumstances in which they are used under close physician supervision. Every time you are prescribed a medication, ask your doctor if that medicine contains a beta-blocker.

Other medications asthmatics should avoid include aspirin and nonsteroidal, anti-inflammatory drugs (NSAIDs), especially if there is a history of nasal polyps (fleshy growths in the nose). Asthmatics with nasal polyps have a high risk of experiencing potentially fatal asthma attacks when exposed to these drugs. Aspirin and NSAID-containing preparations include Actiprofen, Advil, Aleve, Anaprox, Ancasal, Aspergum, ASA, Ascriptin, Azdone, Bayer, Bufferin, Darvon, EC-Naprosyn, Ecotrin, Empirin, Fiorinal, Genprin, IBU, Ibuprin, ibuprofen, Ibuprohm, Magnaprin, Motrin, Naprelan, Naprosyn, naproxen, Naxen, Norwich Extra-Strength, Nuprin, Percodan, St. Joseph Children's Aspirin, Saleto, Synalgos-DC, Synflex, Supasa, and Vicoprofen. If you've been using aspirin or NSAIDs for years without difficulties, ask your doctor if you should still take these medications. If you don't take aspirin or NSAIDs, now is not the time to start, unless you have permission from your physician. Avoid these medications if you have a history of nasal polyps or are known to be sensitive to aspirin or NSAIDs.

IMMUNOTHERAPY

Immunotherapy (or desensitization) involves repeated injection of allergen extracts to desensitize an individual to that allergen. While the mechanisms behind immunotherapy remain a subject of debate, the procedure can help people with allergic rhinitis, allergic asthma, or a history of insect-sting hypersensitivity. Immunotherapy can also be beneficial for asthmatics who have persistent exposure to a known trigger, such as pollen or dust mites. The procedure is, however, not without its risks; people can experience allergic, or potentially life-threatening anaphylactic, reactions to immunotherapy. Another drawback is that immunotherapy often takes, at a minimum, four to five years to complete. Furthermore, once the therapy is finished, the duration of benefit cannot be predicted. Some patients may actually experience a worsening of symptoms once therapy is completed, thereby necessitating the resumption of injections. Many people also find the injections painful. While immunotherapy sounds great, results are mixed at best. Talk to an allergy specialist to learn if immunotherapy is right for you.

FUNDAMENTAL PRINCIPLES OF ASTHMA THERAPY

Underlying all of these medications and procedures is the knowledge that the avoidance of known asthma triggers will always offer asthmatics the most benefit. At their best, drugs represent a second line of defense. No matter what form of therapy you employ, be it a powerful steroid or a humble multivitamin and mineral supplement, it is imperative that you develop a trusting relationship with a knowledgeable healthcare professional.

Equally important is learning to appreciate the severity of your asthma and keeping accurate records of your symptoms and peak flows, which can help guide management. When all is said and done, the best asthma treatment is still healthy living combined with source control. If you follow these simple principles, you can live a long and productive life, without dependence on asthma medications.

Afterword

THERE IS ONE MESSAGE I'D LIKE you to take from this book: You control not only your asthma but your entire life as well. Good health in our increasingly toxic environment is not a passive process but requires active participation. I hope this book has helped you understand how your environment contributes to your asthma. By "environment," I mean not only what's in your home or workplace, but also the environment you create by your eating, sleeping, and exercise habits.

On the surface, asthma may seem like a simple lung problem. After reading this book, however, it should be clear that, for many people, their asthma has to do with how they live. For some people, their diet may be to blame. For others, allergies or air pollution may be the leading factor. Some people may learn that they don't even have asthma; rather, another medical condition is causing their symptoms.

I also hope you now realize that asthma is preventable in many cases. This is why it is so important to go through your home and make a list of asthma triggers and remove these items from your environment. Without question, source control remains the most effective asthma treatment. Supplements, herbs, alternative therapies, and pharmaceuticals are, at best, second-line therapies.

Bottom line: Take control of your asthma, don't let your asthma take control of you. Use the advice in this book to make your home and life healthier. While a healthy diet together with judicious use of supplements can help add years to your life, overall healthy living is most important. Healthy living involves embracing a nutritious diet, adequate sleep, regular exercise, and a balanced, positive outlook toward life. In addition to helping you beat asthma and avoid illnesses such as diabetes, hypertension, and heart disease, healthy living will enable you to enjoy many active and trouble-free decades. You will not only overcome your asthma, but you'll also become the master of your own destiny and enjoy the symptom-free life you so richly deserve.

Notes

Chapter 1: Relax—You're Not Going to Die of Asthma

1. Measuring childhood asthma prevalence before and after the 1997 redesign of the National Health Survey—United States. MMWR 2000;49: 908–911.

2. J.E. Moorman and D.M. Mannino, "Increasing U.S. Asthma Mortality Rates: Who is Really Dying?" *Journal of Asthma,* 38 (2001): 65–71.

3. B.B. Moore, R. Wagner, and K.B. Weiss, "A Community Based Study of Near-fatal Asthma," *Annals of Allergy Asthma Immunology,* 86 (2001): 190–195.

4. A.M. Tatum, et al., "Clinical, Pathologic, and Toxicologic Findings in Asthma Deaths in Cook County, Illinois." *Allergy Asthma Proceedings,* 22 (2001): 285–291.

5. M.O. Turner, K. Noertjojo, S. Vedal, et al., "Risk Factors for Near-fatal Asthma: A Case-control Study in Hospitalized Patients with Asthma," *American Journal of Respiratory and Critical Care Medicine,* 157 (1998): 1804–1809.

6. Nissman, C. Teaming up against asthma: breathing disorder doesn't have to put athletes on sidelines, experts say. 12 March 2001, Boston Herald.com Lifestyle.

7. E. Braundwald, et al., *Harrison's Principles of Internal Medicine,* 15th Edition (New York: McGraw-Hill, 2001), 1463.

8. Ibid.

9. M.D. Silverstein, et al., "Long-term Survival of a Cohort of Community Residents with Asthma," *New England Journal of Medicine,* 331 (1994): 1537–1541.

Chapter 2: Asthma Basics

1. E. Braunwald, A.S. Fauci, D.L. Kasper, et al., *Harrison's Principles of Internal Medicine,* 15th Edition (New York: McGraw-Hill, 2001), 1456.

2. H. Yemaneberhan, Z. Bekele, A. Venn, et al., "Prevalence of Wheeze and Asthma and Relation to Atopy in Urban and Rural Ethiopia," *The Lancet,* 350 (1997): 85–90.

3. C.H. Van Niekerk, E.G. Weinberg, S.C. Shore, et al., "Prevalence of Asthma in Xhosa Children: A Comparative Study of Urban and Rural Xhosa Children," *Clinical Allergy,* 9 (1979): 319–324.

4. M. Cluzel, M. Damon, P. Chanez, et al., "Enhanced Alveolar Cell Luminol-dependent Chemiluminescence in Asthma," *Journal of Allergy and Clinical Immunology,* 80 (1987): 195–201.

5. B.S. Jonas, D.K. Wagener, J.J. Lando, et al., "Symptoms of Anxiety and Depression as a Risk Factor for the Development of Asthma," *Journal of Applied Biobehavioral Research,* 4 (1999): 91–110.

6. B.A. Aba-Alkhail and F.M. El-Gamal, "Prevalence of Food Allergy in Asthmatic Patients," *Saudi Medical Journal,* 21 (2000): 81–87.

7. K.A. Ogle and J.D. Bullock, "Children with Allergic Rhinitis and/or Bronchial Asthma Treated with Elimination Diet," *Annals of Allergy,* 39 (1977): 8–11.

8. J.M. James, "Food Allergy and the Respiratory Tract," *Current Allergy Reports,* 1 (2001): 54–60.

9. Y.I. Koh and S. Choi, "Blood Eosinophil Counts for the Predication of the Severity of Exercise-induced Bronchospasm in Asthma," *Respiratory Medicine,* 96 (2002): 120–125.

10. T. Gislason, C. Janson, P. Vermeire, et al., "Respiratory Symptoms and Nocturnal Gastroesophageal Reflux: A Population-based Study of Young Adults in Three European Countries," *Chest,* 121 (2002): 158–163.

11. H.R. Foroutan and M. Ghafari, "Gastroesophageal Reflux as a Cause of Chronic Respiratory Symptoms," *Indian Journal of Pediatrics,* 69 (2002): 137–139.

12. F. Cibella and G. Cuttitta, "Nocturnal Asthma and Gastroesophageal Reflux," *American Journal of Medicine,* 111 (2001): 31S–36S.

13. M. Perrin-Fayolle, F. Gormand, G. Braillon, et al., "Long-term Results of Surgical Treatment for Gastroesophageal Reflux in Asthmatic Patients," *Chest,* 96 (1989): 40–45.

14. T.M. Farrell, W.S. Richardson, T.L. Trus, et al., "Response of Atypical Symptoms of Gastroesophageal Reflux to Antireflux Surgery," *British Journal of Surgery,* 88 (2001): 1649–1652.

15. M. Ribet, F.R. Pruvot, E. Mensier, et al., "Gastro-oesophageal Reflux and Respiratory Disorders Treated by Hill's Procedure," *European Journal of Cardiothoracic Surgery,* 3 (1989): 414–417.

Chapter 3: What Type of Asthmatic Are You?

1. G. Bronfort, R.L. Evans, P. Kubic, et al., "Chronic Pediatric Asthma and Chiropractic Spinal Manipulation: A Prospective Clinical Series and Randomized Clinical Pilot Study," *Journal of Manipulative Physiologic Therapy,* 24 (2001): 369–377.

Chapter 4: Healthy Living Boot Camp I—You Are What You Eat

1. E. Ernst, "Complementary Therapies for Asthma: What Patients Use," *Journal of Asthma,* 35 (1998): 667–671.

2. Ibid.

3. P.G.J. Burney, "A Diet Rich in Sodium May Potentate Asthma: Epidemiological Evidence for a New Hypothesis," *Chest,* 91 Suppl. (1987): 143S–148S.

4. A. Soutar, A. Seaton, and K. Brown, "Bronchial Reactivity and Dietary Antioxidants," *Thorax,* 52 (1997): 166–170.

5. F. Forastiere, R. Pistelli, P. Sestini, et al., "Consumption of Fresh Fruit Rich in Vitamin C and Wheezing Symptoms in Children," *Thorax,* 55 (2000): 3283–3288.

6. D.G. Cook, I.M. Carey, P.H. Whincup, et al., "Effect of Fresh Fruit Consumption on Lung Function and Wheeze in Children," *Thorax,* 52 (1997): 628–633.

7. D.P. Strachen, B.D. Cox, S.W. Erzinclioglu, et al., "Ventilatory Function and Winter Fresh Fruit Consumption in a Random Sample of British Adults," *Thorax,* 46 (1991): 624–629.

8. P. Ellwood, M.I. Asher, B. Bjorksten, et al., "Diet and Asthma, Allergic Rhinoconjunctivitis and Atopic Eczema Symptoms Prevalence: An Ecological Analysis of the International Study of Asthma and Allergic Childhood (ISAAC) Data, ISAAC Phase One Study Group," *European Respiratory Journal,* 17 (2001): 436–443.

9. I. Neuman, H. Nahum, and A. Ben-Amotz, "Prevention of Exercise-induced Asthma by a Natural Isomer Mixture of Beta-carotene," *Annals of Allergy, Asthma, and Immunology,* 82 (1999): 549–553.

10. I. Neuman, H. Nahum, and A. Ben-Amotz, "Reduction in Exercise-induced Asthma Oxidative Stress by Lycopene, a Natural Antioxidant," *Allergy,* 55 (2000): 1184–1189.

11. S.O. Shaheen, J.A. Sterne, R.L. Thompson, et al., "Dietary Antioxidants and Asthma in Adults: Population-based Case-control Study," *American Journal of Respiratory and Critical Care Medicine,* 15 (2001): 1823–1828.

12. A. Fogarty, and J. Britton, "The Role of Diet in the Etiology of Asthma," *Clinical and Experimental Allergy,* 30 (2000): 615–627.

13. F.B. Hu, L. Bronner, W.C. Willett, et al., "Fish and Omega-3 Fatty Acid Intake and Risk of Coronary Heart Disease in Women," *Journal of the American Medical Association,* 287 (2002): 1815–1821.

14. L. Hodge, C.M. Salome, J.K. Peat, et al., "Consumption of Oily Fish and Childhood Asthma Risk," *Medical Journal of Australia,* 164 (1996): 137–140.

15. J. Schwartz, and S.T. Weiss, "The Relationship of Dietary Fish Intake to Level of Pulmonary Function in the First National Health and Nutrition Survey (NHANES 1)," *European Respiratory Journal,* 7 (1994): 1821–1824.

16. J. Schwartz, "Role of Polyunsaturated Fatty Acids in Lung Disease," *American Journal of Clinical Nutrition,* 71 (2000): S393–S396.

17. F. Villani, R. Comazzi, P. DeMaria, et al., "Effect of Dietary Supplementation with Polyunsaturated Fatty Acids on Bronchial Hyperreactivity in Subjects with Seasonal Asthma," *Respiration,* 65 (1998): 265–269.

18. K. Strom, L. Janzon, I. Mattisson, et al., "Asthma but Not Smoking-related Airflow Limitation is Associated with High-fat Diet in Men: Results from the Population Study 'Men Born in 1914,' Malmo, Sweden," *Monaldi Archives of Chest Disease,* 51 (1996): 16–21.

19. S.L. Huang, and W.H. Pan, "Dietary Fats and Asthma in Teenagers: Analysis of the First Nutrition and Health Survey in Taiwan (NAHSIT)," *Clinical and Experimental Allergy,* 31 (2001): 1875–1880.

20. O. Lindahl, L. Lindwall, A. Spangberg, et al., "Vegan Regimen with Reduced Medication in the Treatment of Bronchial Asthma," *Journal of Asthma,* 22 (1985): 45–55.

21. J. Schwartz, and S.T. Weiss, "Caffeine Intake and Asthma Symptoms," *Annals of Epidemiology,* 2 (1992): 627–635.

22. R.E. Pagano, E. Negri, A. Decarli, et al., "Coffee Drinking and Prevalence of Bronchial Asthma," *Chest,* 94 (1988): 386–389.

23. S. Kivity, A.Y. Ben, A. Man, et al., "The Effect of Caffeine on Exercise-induced Bronchoconstriction," *Chest,* 97 (1990): 1083–1085.

24. M. Bukowskyj, and K. Nakatsu, "The Bronchodilator Effect of Caffeine in Adult Asthmatics," *American Review of Respiratory Disease,* 135 (1987): 173–175.

25. A.I. Bara, and E.A. Barley, "Caffeine for Asthma," *Cochrane Database Systematic Review,* 4 (2001): CD001112.

26. R. Pistelli, F. Forastiere, G.M. Corbo, et al., "Respiratory Symptoms and Bronchial Responsiveness are Related to Dietary Salt Intake and Urinary Potassium Excretion in Male Children," *European Respiratory Journal,* 6 (1993): 517–522.

27. K.D. Ardern and F.S.F. Ram, "Dietary Salt Reduction or Exclusion for Allergic Asthma," In: *The Cochrane Library, Issue 1* (Oxford: Update Software, 2002).

28. T.D. Mickleborough, R.W. Gotshall, L. Cordain, et al., "Dietary Salt Alters Pulmonary Function During Exercise in Exercise-induced Asthma," *Journal of Sports Science,* 19 (2001): 865–873.

29. T.D. Mickleborough, R.W. Gotshall, E.M. Kluka, et al., "Dietary Chloride as a Possible Determinant of the Severity of Exercise-induced Asthma," *European Journal of Applied Physiology,* 85 (2001): 450–456.

Chapter 5: Healthy Living Boot Camp II—Exercise, Sleep, and Eliminating Bad Habits

1. W. Nystad, J. Harris, and J.S. Borgen, "Asthma and Wheezing Among Norwegian Elite Athletes," *Medicine Science and Sports Exercise,* 32 (2000): 266–270.

2. I. Helenius, and T. Haahtela, "Allergy and Asthma in Elite Summer Sport Athletes," *Journal of Asthma and Clinical Immunology,* 106 (2000): 444–452.

3. I. Helenius, and T. Haahtela, "Allergy and Asthma in Elite Summer Sport Athletes," *Journal of Asthma and Clinical Immunology,* 106 (2000): 444–452.

4. L.A. Sonna, K.C. Angel, M.A. Sharp, et al., "The Prevalence of Exercise-induced Bronchospasm Among U.S. Army Recruits and Its Effects on Physical Performance," *Chest,* 119 (2001): 1676–1684.

5. A. Satta, "Exercise Training in Asthma," *Journal of Sports Medicine and Physical Fitness,* 40 (2000): 277–283.

6. J.A. Neder, L.E. Nery, A.C. Silva, et al., "Short-term Effects of Aerobic Training in the Clinical Management of Moderate to Severe Asthma in Children," *Thorax,* 54 (1999): 202–206.

7. M. Emtner, M. Finne, and G. Stalenheim, "High-intensity Physical Training in Adults with Asthma: A Comparison Between Training on Land and in Water," *Scandinavian Journal of Rehabilitation Medicine,* 30 (1998): 201–209.

8. R.M. Bingisser, L. Joos, B. Fruhauf, et al., "Pulmonary Rehabilitation in Outpatients with Asthma or Chronic Obstructive Lung Disease: A Pilot Study of a 'Modular' Rehabilitation Program," *Swiss Medical Weekly,* 131 (2001): 407–411.

9. M. Emtner, M. Finne, and G. Stalenheim, "A 3-year Follow-up of Asthmatic Patients Participating in a 10-week Rehabilitation Program with Emphasis on Physical Training," *Archives of Physical Medicine and Rehabilitation,* 79 (1998): 539–544.

10. M. Zsiray, M. Dervaderics, and A. Toth, "The Effect of Conditioning Inhaled Air in Exercise-induced Asthma," *Allergy Immunology,* (Leipzig) 29 (1983): 212–214.

11. Y. Chen, R. Dales, M. Tang, et al., "Obesity May Increase the Incidence of Asthma in Women but Not in Men: Longitudinal Observations from the Canadian National Population Healthy Surveys," *American Journal of Epidemiology,* 155 (2002): 191–197.

12. W.S. Beckett, D.R. Jacobs, X. Yu, et al., "Asthma is Associated with Weight Gain in Females but Not in Males, Independent of Physical Activity," *American Journal of Respiratory and Critical Care Medicine,* 164 (2001): 2045–2050.

13. J.C. Celedon, L.J. Palmer, A.A. Litonjua, et al., "Body Mass Index and Asthma in Adults in Families of Subjects with Asthma in Anqing, China," *American Journal of Respiratory Critical Care Medicine,* 164 (2001): 1835–1840.

14. G. Stores, A.J. Ellis, L. Wigs, et al., "Sleep and Psychological Disturbance in Nocturnal Asthma," *Archives of Diseases in Children,* 78 (1998): 413–419.

15. S.O. Shaheen, J.A. Sterne, R.L. Thompson, et al., "Dietary Antioxidants and Asthma in Adults: Population-based Case-control Study," *American Journal of Respiratory and Critical Care Medicine,* 15 (2001): 1823–1828.

Chapter 6: Home Decorating for the Asthmatic

1. Environmental Protection Agency, *The Inside Story: A Guide to Indoor Air Quality,* EPA 402-K-93-007 (Washington, DC: U.S. EPA, U.S. CPSC, April 1995). Available at the EPA website: www.epa.gov/iaq/pubs/insidest.html.

2. H.S. Nelson, S.R. Hirsh, J.L. Ohman, et al., "Recommendations of the Use of Residential Air Cleaning Devices in the Treatment of Allergic Respiratory Diseases," *Journal of Allergy and Clinical Immunology,* 82 (1988): 661–669.

3. Environmental Protection Agency, *Ozone Generators That are Sold as Air Cleaners: An Assessment of Effectiveness and Health Consequences,* (Washington, DC: U.S. EPA, U.S. CPSC). Available on the EPA website: www.epa.gov/iaq/pubs/ozonegen.html.

4. H.S. Nelson, S.R. Hirsh, J.L. Ohman, et al., "Recommendations of the Use of Residential Air Cleaning Devices in the Treatment of Allergic Respiratory Diseases," *Journal of Allergy and Clinical Immunology,* 82 (1988): 661–669.

5. C.J. Warburton, R.M. Niven, C.A. Pickering, et al., "Domiciliary Air Filtration Units, Symptoms and Lung Function in Atopic Asthmatics," *Respiratory Medicine,* 88 (1994): 771–776.

6. H. Harving, J. Korsgaard, and R. Dahl, "House Dust Mite Exposure Reduction in Specially Designed, Mechanically Ventilated 'Healthy' Homes," *Allergy,* 49 (1994): 713–718.

7. T.J. Lintner, and K.A. Brame, "The Effects of Season, Climate, and Air-conditioning on the Prevalence of *Dermatophagoides* Mite Allergens in Household Dust," *Journal of Allergy and Clinical Immunology,* 91 (1993): 862–867.

8. J.K. Peat, E. Tovey, B.G. Toelle, et al., "House Dust Mite Allergens: A Major Risk Factor for Childhood Asthma in Australia," *American Journal of Respiratory Care,* 153 (1996): 141–146.

9. E. Bjornsson, D. Norback, C. Janson, et al., "Asthmatic Symptoms and Indoor Levels of Microorganisms and House Dust Mites," *Clinical Experimental Allergy,* 25 (1995): 423–431.

10. E.J. Popplewell, V.A. Innes, S. Lloyd-Hughes, et al., "The Effect of High-efficiency and Standard Vacuum-cleaners on Mite, Cat and Dog Allergen Levels and Clinical Progress," *Pediatric Allergy and Immunology,* 11 (2000): 142–148.

11. J.A. Warner, J.M. Frederick, T.N. Bryant, et al., "Mechanical Ventilation and High-efficiency Vacuum Cleaning: A Combined Strategy of Mite and Mite Allergen Reduction in the Control of Mite-sensitive Asthma," *Journal of Allergy and Clinical Immunology,* 105 (2000): 75–82.

12. P.J. Vojta, S.P. Randels, J. Stout, et al., "Effects of Physical Interventions on House Dust Mite Allergen Levels in Carpet, Bed, and Upholstery Dust in Low-income, Urban Homes," *Environmental Health Perspectives,* 109 (2001): 815–819.

13. T. Htut, T.W. Higenbottam, G.W. Gill, et al., "Eradication of House Dust Mite from Homes of Atopic Asthmatics Subjects: A Double-blind Trial," *Journal of Allergy and Clinical Immunology,* 107 (2001): 55–60.

14. Environmental Protection Agency, *The Inside Story: A Guide to Indoor Air Quality,* EPA 402-K-93-007 (Washington, DC: U.S. EPA, U.S. CPSC, April 1995). Available at the EPA website: www.epa.gov/iaq/pubs/insidest.html.

15. B. Ehnert, S. Lau-Schadendorf, A. Weber, et al., "Reducing Domestic Exposure to Dust Mite Allergen Reduces Bronchial Hyperreactivity in Sensitive Children with Asthma," *Journal of Allergy and Clinical Immunology,* 90 (1992): 135–138.

16. A.B. Murray and A.C. Ferguson, "Dust Free Bedrooms in the Treatment of Asthmatic Children with House Dust or House Dust Mite Allergy: A Randomized Controlled Trial," *Pediatrics,* 71 (1983): 418–422.

17. S.H. Arshad, S. Matthews, C. Gant, et al., "Effect of Allergen Avoidance on Development of Allergic Disorders in Infancy," *The Lancet,* 339 (1992): 1493–1497.

18. D.W. Hide, S. Matthews, L. Matthews, et al., "Effect of Allergen Avoidance in Infancy on Allergic Manifestations at Age Two Years," *Journal of Allergy and Clinical Immunology,* 93 (1993): 842–846.

19. D.L. Rosenstreich, P. Eggleston, M. Kattan, et al., "The Role of Cockroach Allergy and Exposure to Cockroach Allergen in Causing Morbidity Among Inner-city Children with Asthma," *New England Journal of Medicine,* 336 (1997): 1356–1363.

20. T. Hodson, A. Custovic, A. Simpson, et al., "Washing the Dog Reduces Dog Allergen Levels, but the Dog Needs to Be Washed Twice a Week," *Journal of Allergy and Clinical Immunology,* (1999): 581–585.

21. P. Plaschke, C. Janson, B. Balder, et al., "Adult Asthmatics Sensitized to Cats and Dogs: Symptoms, Severity, and Bronchial Hyperresponsiveness in Patients with Furred Animals at Home and Patients Without These Animals," *Allergy,* 54 (1999): 843–850.

22. Environmental Protection Agency, *The Inside Story: A Guide to Indoor Air Quality,* EPA 402-K-93-007 (Washington, DC: U.S. EPA, U.S. CPSC, April 1995). Available at the EPA website: www.epa.gov/iaq/pubs/insidest.html.

Chapter 7: Vitamin, Mineral, and Dietary Supplements

1. S.E. McGowan, J. Smith, A.J. Holms, et al., "Vitamin A Deficiency Promotes Bronchial Hyperreactivity in Rates by Altering Muscarinic M(2) Receptor Function," *American Journal of Physiology and Lung Cellular Molecular Physiology,* 282 (2002): 1031–1039.

2. A. Morabia, M.J.S. Menkes, C.W. Comstock, et al., "Serum Retinol and Airway Obstruction," *American Journal of Epidemiology,* 132 (1990): 77–82.

3. M.S. Tockman, M.J. Khoury, and B.H. Cohen, "Milk Drinking and Possible Protection of the Respiratory Epithelium," *Journal of Chronic Disease,* 39 (1986): 207–209.

4. A. Morabia, A. Sorenson, S. Kumanyiki, et al., "Vitamin A, Cigarette Smoking, and Airway Obstruction," *American Review of Respiratory Disease,* 140 (1989): 1312–1316.

5. J.C. Baker, W.S. Tunnicliffe, R.C. Duncanson, et al., "Dietary Antioxidants and Magnesium in Type 1 Brittle Asthma: A Case Control Study," *Thorax,* 54 (1999): 115–118.

6. J.A. Denburg, R. Sehmi, and J. Upham, "Regulation of IL-5 Receptor on Eosinophils Progenitors in Allergic Inflammation: Role of Retinoic Acid," *International Archives of Allergy and Immunology,* 124 (2001): 246–248.

7. T. Shimizu, S. Maeda, H. Arakawa, et al., "Relation Between Theophylline and Circulating Vitamin Levels in Children with Asthma," *Pharmacology,* 53 (1996): 384–389.

8. M. Garcia and R. Gonzalez, "Effect on Pyridoxine on Histamine Liberation and Degranulation of Rat Mast Cells," *Allergol Immunopathol,* 7 (1979): 427–432.

9. E. Bikier, J. Wyczolkowska, H. Szye, et al., "The Inhibitory Effect of Nicotinamide on Asthma-like Symptoms and Eosinophilia in Guinea Pigs, Anaphylactic Mast Cell Degranulation in Mice, and Histamine Release from Rat Isolated Peritoneal Mast Cells by Compound 48–80," *International Archives of Allergy and Applied Immunology,* 47 (1974): 737–748.

10. J. Schwartz and S.T. Weiss, "Dietary Factors and Their Relation to Respiratory Symptoms: The Second National Health and Nutrition Examination Survey," *American Journal of Epidemiology,* 132 (1990): 67–76.

11. Z. Czezowska, B. Kowal-Gierczak, and M. Wrzyszcz, "The Effect of Nicotinamide on the Urinary 17-hydroxysteroid Excretion in Patients with Allergic Bronchial Asthma," *Polish Medical Journal,* 10 (1971): 42–46.

12. E.M. Rozanov, L.K. Iutanova, A.P. Podorozhnyi, et al., "Vitamin P and C Allowances and Their Correction in the Treatment of Bronchial Asthma Patients," *Vopr Pitan,* 6 (1987): 21–24.

13. R.D. Reynolds and C.L. Natta, "Depressed Plasma Pyridoxal Phosphate Concentrations in Adult Asthmatics," *American Journal of Clinical Nutrition,* 41 (1985): 684–688.

14. T. Shimizu, S. Maeda, H. Arakawa, et al., "Relation Between Theophylline and Circulating Vitamin Levels in Children with Asthma," *Pharmacology,* 53 (1996): 384–389.

15. P.J. Collipp, S. Goldzier, N. Weiss, et al., "Pyridoxine Treatment of Childhood Bronchial Asthma," *Annals of Allergy,* 35 (1975): 93–97.

16. R.D. Reynolds and C.L. Natta, "Depressed Plasma Pyridoxal Phosphate Concentrations in Adult Asthmatics," *American Journal of Clinical Nutrition,* 41 (1985): 684–688.

17. R.G. Alvarez and M.G. Mesa, "Ascorbic Acid and Pyridoxine in Experimental Anaphylaxis," *Agents and Actions,* 11 (1981): 89–93.

18. S. Sur, M. Camara, A. Buchmeier, et al., "Double-blind Trial of Pyridoxine (Vitamin B_6) in the Treatment of Steroid-dependent Asthma," *Annals of Allergy,* 70 (1993): 147–152.

19. B. Anibarro, T. Caballero, C. Garcia-Ara, et al., "Asthma with Sulfite Intolerance in Children: A Blocking Study with Cyanocobalamin," *Journal of Allergy and Clinical Immunology,* 90 (1992): 130–139.

20. C. Bucca, G.A. Rolla, and W. Arossa, "Effect of Ascorbic Acid on Increased Bronchial Responsiveness During Upper Airway Infection," *Respiration,* 55 (1989): 214–219.

21. C.S. Johnston, K.R. Retrum, and J.C. Srilakshmi, "Antihistamine Effects and Complications of Supplementing Vitamin C," *Journal of the American Dietary Association,* 92 (1992): 988–989.

22. G.E. Hatch, "Asthma, Inhaled Oxidants, and Dietary Antioxidants," *American Journal of Clinical Nutrition,* 61 (1995): 625S–630S.

23. J. Schwartz and S.T. Weiss, "Relationship Between Dietary Vitamin C Intake and Pulmonary Function in the First National Health and Nutrition Examination Survey (NHANES I)," *American Journal of Clinical Nutrition,* 59 (1994): 110–114.

24. S.L. Huang and W.H. Pan, "Dietary Fats and Asthma in Teenagers: Analysis of the First Nutrition and Health Survey in Taiwan (NAHSIT)," *Clinical Experimental Allergy,* 31 (2001): 1875–1880.

25. V. Mohsenin, "Effect of Vitamin C on NO2-induced Airway Hyperresponsiveness in Normal Subjects: A Randomized Double-blind Experiment," *American Review of Respiratory Disease,* 136 (1987): 1408–1411.

26. V. Mohsenin, A.B. Dubois, and J.S. Douglas, "Effect of Ascorbic Acid on Response to Methacholine Challenge in Asthmatic Subjects," *American Review of Respiratory Disease,* 127 (1983): 143–147.

27. A. Soutar, A. Seaton, and K. Brown, "Bronchial Reactivity and Dietary Antioxidants," *Thorax,* 52 (1997): 166–170.

28. C.O. Anah, L.N. Jariek, and H.A. Baig, "High-dose Ascorbic Acid in Nigerian Asthmatics," *Tropical Geographic Medicine,* 32 (1980): 132–137.

29. D.G. Cook, I.M. Carey, P.H. Whincup, et al., "Effect of Fruit Consumption on Lung Function and Wheeze in Children," *Thorax,* 52 (1997): 628–633.

30. F. Forastiere, R. Pistelli, P. Sestini, et al., "Consumption of Fresh Fruit Rich in Vitamin C and Wheezing Symptoms in Children," *Thorax,* 55 (2000): 3283–288.

31. D.P. Strachan, B.D. Cox, S.W. Erzinclioglu, et al., "Ventilatory Function and Winter Fresh Fruit Consumption in a Random Sample of British Adults," *Thorax,* 46 (1991): 624–629.

32. B.K. Butland, D.P. Strachan, and H.R. Anderson, "Fresh Fruit Intake and Asthma Symptoms in Young British Adults: Confounding or Effect Modification by Smoking?" *European Respiratory Journal,* 13 (1999): 744–750.

33. E.N. Schachter and A. Schlesinger, "The Attenuation of Exercise-induced Bronchospasm by Ascorbic Acid," *Annals of Allergy,* 49 (1982): 146–151.

34. H.A. Cohen, I. Neuman, and H. Nahum, "Blocking Effect of Vitamin C in Exercise-induced Asthma," *Archives of Pediatric and Adolescent Medicine,* 151 (1997): 367–370.

35. E.M. Peters, J.M. Goetzsche, et al., "Vitamin C Supplementation Reduces the Incidence of Post-race Symptoms of Upper-respiratory-tract Infection in Ultra-marathon Runners," *American Journal of Clinical Nutrition,* 57 (1993): 170–174.

36. G. Utz and A.M. Hauck, "Oral Application of Calcium and Vitamin D2 in Allergic Bronchial Asthma," *Munch Med Wochenschr,* 118 (1976): 1395–1398.

37. E.B. Rimm, M.J. Stampfer, A. Ascherio, et al., "Vitamin E Consumption and the Risk of Coronary Heart Disease in Men," *New England Journal of Medicine,* 328 (1993): 1450–1456. See also: M.J. Stampfer, C.H. Hennekens, J.E. Manson, et al., "Vitamin E Consumption and the Risk of Coronary Heart Disease in Women," *New England Journal of Medicine,* 328 (1993): 1444–1449.

38. A. Fogarty, S. Lewis, S. Weiss, et al., "Dietary Vitamin E Concentrations, and Atopy," *The Lancet,* 356 (2000): 1573–1574.

39. S.N. Meydani, M. Meydani, J.B. Blumberg, et al., "Vitamin E Supplementation and *in vivo* Immune Response in Healthy Elderly Subjects," *Journal of the American Medical Association,* 227 (1997): 1380–1386.

40. E.B. Pallast, E.G. Schouten, F.G. de Waart, et al., "Effect of 50- and 100-mg Vitamin E Supplementation on Cellular Immune Function in Non-institutionalized Elderly Persons," *American Journal of Clinical Nutrition,* 69 (1999): 1273–1281.

41. M.D. Chatham, J.H. Eppler, L.R. Sauder, et al., "Evaluation of the Effects of Vitamin C on Ozone-induced Bronchoconstriction in Normal Subjects," *Annals of the New York Academy of Sciences,* 498 (1987): 269–279.

42. C. Bodner, D. Godden, K. Brown, et al., "Antioxidant Intake and Adult-onset Wheeze: A Case-control Study. Aberdeen WHEASE Study Group," *European Respiratory Journal,* 13 (1999): 22–30.

43. L. Dow, M. Tracy, A. Villar, et al., "Does Dietary Intake of Vitamins C and E Influence Lung Function in Older People?" *American Journal Respiratory Critical Care Medicine,* 154 (1996): 1401–1404.

44. R.J. Troisi, W.C. Willett, S.T. Weiss, et al., "A Prospective Study of Diet and Adult-onset Asthma," *American Journal of Respiratory and Critical Care Medicine,* 151 (1995): 1401–1408.

45. J.C. Baker, W.S. Tunnicliffe, R.C. Duncanson, et al., "Dietary Antioxidants and Magnesium in Type 1 Brittle Asthma: A Case Control Study," *Thorax,* 54 (1999): 115–118.

46. A. Fogarty, S. Lewis, S. Weiss, et al., "Dietary Vitamin E Concentrations and Atopy," *The Lancet,* 356 (2000): 1573–1574.

47. H.R. De Raeve, F.B. Thunnissen, F.T. Kaneko, et al., "Decreased Cu,Zn-SOD Activity in Asthmatic Airway Epithelium: Correction by Inhaled Corticosteroid *in vivo,*" *American Journal of Physiology,* 272 (1997): L148–154.

48. J. Schwartz, and S.T. Weiss, "Dietary Factors and Their Relation to Respiratory Symptoms: The Second National Health and Nutrition Examination Survey," *American Journal of Epidemiology,* 132 (1990): 67–76.

49. D. Sparrow, J. Silbert, and S. Weiss, "The Relationship of Pulmonary Function to Copper Concentrations in Drinking Water," *American Review of Respiratory Disease,* 126 (1982): 312–315.

50. L.A. Macmillan-Crow and D.L. Cruthirds, "Invited Review: Manganese Superoxide Dismutase in Disease," *Free Radical Research,* 34 (2001): 325–336.

51. A. Soutar, A. Seaton, and K. Brown, "Bronchial Reactivity and Dietary Antioxidants," *Thorax,* 52 (1997): 166–170.

52. O.S. Alamoudi, "Hypomagnesemia in Chronic, Stable Asthmatics: Prevalence, Correlation with Severity and Hospitalization," *European Respiratory Journal,* 16 (2000): 427–431.

53. L.J. Dominguez, M. Barbagallo, G. Di Lorenzo, et al., "Bronchial Reactivity and Intracellular Magnesium: A Possible Mechanism for the Bronchodilating Effect of Magnesium in Asthma," *Clinical Science,* 95 (1998): 137–142.

54. A. Soutar, A. Seaton, and K. Brown, "Bronchial Reactivity and Dietary Antioxidants," *Thorax,* 52 (1997): 166–170.

55. J.C. Baker, W.S. Tunnicliffe, R.C. Duncanson, et al., "Dietary Antioxidants and Magnesium in Type 1 Brittle Asthma: A Case-control Study," *Thorax,* 54 (1999): 115–118.

56. J. Britton, I. Pavord, K. Richards, et al., "Dietary Magnesium, Lung Function, Wheezing, and Airway Hyperreactivity in a Random Adult Population Sample," *The Lancet,* 334 (1994): 357–362.

57. J. Hill, A. Micklewright, S. Lewis, et al., "Investigation of the Effect of Short-term Change in Dietary Magnesium Intake in Asthma," *European Respiratory Journal,* 10 (1997): 2225–2229.

58. L.C. Clark, G.F. Combs, B.W. Turnbull, et al., "Effects of Selenium Supplementation for Cancer Prevention in Patients with Carcinoma of the Skin," *Journal of the American Medical Association,* 276 (1996): 1957–1963.

59. A. Flatt, N. Pearce, C.D. Thomson, et al., "Reduced Selenium in Asthmatic Subjects in New Zealand," *Thorax,* 45 (1990): 95–99.

60. L. Hasselmark, R. Malmgren, O. Zatterstrom, et al., "Selenium Supplementation in Intrinsic Asthma," *Allergy,* 48 (1993): 30–36.

61. S.O. Shaheen, J.A. Sterne, R.L. Thompson, et al., "Dietary Antioxidants and Asthma in Adults: Population-based Case-control Study," *American Journal of Respiratory and Critical Care Medicine,* 15 (2001): 1823–1828.

62. J.C. Baker, W.S. Tunnicliffe, R.C. Duncanson, et al., "Dietary Antioxidants and Magnesium in Type 1 Brittle Asthma: A Case-control Study," *Thorax,* 54 (1999): 115–118.

63. H.R. De Raeve, F.B. Thunnissen, F.T. Kaneko, et al., "Decreased Cu,Zn-SOD Activity in Asthmatic Airway Epithelium: Correction by Inhaled Corticosteroid *in vivo*," *American Journal of Physiology,* 272 (1997): L148–154.

64. A. Soutar, A. Seaton, and K. Brown, "Bronchial Reactivity and Dietary Antioxidants," *Thorax,* 52 (1997): 166–170.

65. P. Cazzola, P. Mazzanti, and G. Bossi, "*In vivo* Modulating Effect of a Calf Thymus Acid Lysate on Human T-lymphocyte Subsets and CD4+/CD8+ Ratio in the Course on Different Diseases," *Current Therapies and Research,* 42 (1987): 1011–1017.

66. N.M. Kouttab, M. Prada, and P. Cazzola, "Thymomodulin: Biological Properties and Clinical Applications," *Med Oncol Tumor Pharmacotherapy,* 6 (1989): 5–9. See also: R. Marzari, P. Mazzanti, P. Cazzola, et al., "Perennial Allergic Rhinitis: Prevention of Acute Episodes with Thymomodulin," *Minerva Med,* 78 (1987): 1675–1681.

67. R. Marzari, P. Mazzanti, P. Cazzola, et al., "Perennial Allergic Rhinitis: Prevention of Acute Episodes with Thymomodulin," *Minerva Med,* 78 (1987): 1675–1681.

68. A. Bagnato, P. Brovedani, P. Comina, et al., "Long-term Treatment with Thymomodulin Reduces Airway Hyperresponsiveness to Methacholine," *Annals of Allergy,* 62 (1989): 425–428.

69. R. Genova and A. Guerra, "Un Estratto di Timo (Timomodulina) Nella Profilassi del'Asma Infantile," *Ped Med Chir,* 5 (1983): 395–402.

Chapter 8: Herbs for Asthma Relief

1. I. Gupta, V. Gupta, A. Parihar, et al., "Effects of *Boswellia serrata* Gum Resin in Patients with Bronchial Asthma: Results of a Double-blind, Placebo-controlled, 6-week Clinical Study," *European Journal of Medical Research,* 3 (1998): 511–514.

2. X. Yuan, X. Ning, and F. Liu, "Clinical and Experimental Study on the Houpu Mahuang Oral Liquid in Treating Bronchial Asthma," *Zhongguo Zhong Xi Yi Za Zhi,* 18 (1998): 517–519.

3 D.S. Xu, Z.Y. Shen, W.J. Wang, et al., "Study on Effect of Strengthening Body Resistance Method on Asthmatic Attack," *Chung Kuo Chine His I Chieh Ho Tsa Chih,* 16 (1996): 198–200.

4. C. Touvay, A. Etienne, and P. Braquet, "Inhibition of Antigen-induced Lung Anaphylaxis in the Guinea-pig by BN 52021: A New Specific Paf-acether Receptor Antagonist Isolated from *Ginkgo biloba,*" *Agents and Actions,* 17 (1986): 371–372.

5. J. Ni, J. Dong, and G. Wu, "Experimental Study on Effect of Antagonizing Platelet-activating Factor and Histamine of Synthetic Ginkgolide F in Guinea-pigs," *Zhongguo Zhong Xi Yi Jie He Za Zhi,* 20 (2000): 365–367.

6. M. Li, H. Zhang, and B. Yang, "Effects of Ginkgo Leaf Concentrated Oral Liquor in Treating Asthma," *Chung Kuo Ching Hsi 1 Chich Ho Tsa Chieh,* 17 (1997): 216–218.

7. H.J. Mansfeld, H. Hohre, R. Repges, et al., "Therapy of Bronchial Asthma with Dried Ivy Leaf," *Munch Med Wschr,* 140 (1998): 26–30. See also: A. Huntley and E. Ernst, "Herbal Medicines for Asthma: A Systematic Review," *Thorax,* 55 (2000): 925–929.

8. D.P. Tashkin, B.J. Shapiro, Y.E. Lee, et al., "Effects of Smoked Marijuana in Experimentally Induced Asthma," *American Review of Respiratory Disease,* 112 (1975): 377–386.

9. D.P. Tashkin, et al., *American Review of Respiratory Disease,* 115 (1977): 57–65.

10. D.P. Tashkin, B.J. Shapiro, and I.M. Frank, "Acute Effects of Marihuana on Airway Dynamics in Spontaneous and Experimentally Induced Bronchial Asthma," In: M.C. Braude and S. Szara, eds., *The Pharmacology of Marihuana,* (New York: Raven Press, 1976), 785–801.

11. G.B. Patrick, "Marijuana and the Lung," *Postgraduate Medicine,* 67 (1980): 110–113.

12. J.R. Stokes, R. Hartel, L.B. Ford, et al., "Cannabis (Hemp) Positive Skin Tests and Respiratory Symptoms," *Annals of Allergy, Asthma, and Immunology,* 85 (2000): 238–240.

13. D.P. Tashkin, J.R. Soares, R.S. Hepler, et al., "Cannabis, 1977," *Annals of Internal Medicine,* 89 (1978): 539–549.

14. D. Bickel, T. Roder, H.J. Bestmann, et al., "Identification and Characterization of Inhibitors of Peptido-leukotriene Synthesis from *Petasites hybridus,*" *Planta Medica,* 60 (1994): 318–322. See also: K. Brune, D. Bickel, and B.A. Peskar, "Gastro-protective Effects by Extracts of *Petasites hybridus:* The Role of Inhibition of Peptido-leukotriene Synthesis," *Planta Medica,* 59 (1993): 494–496.

15. G. Ziolo and L. Samochoweic, "Study on Clinical Properties and Mechanisms of Action of *Petasites* in Bronchial Asthma and Chronic Obstructive Bronchitis," *Pharm Acta Helv,* 72 (1998): 378–380.

16. I. Kobayashi, Y. Hamasaki, R. Sato, et al., "Saiboku-To, an Herbal Extract Mixture, Selectively Inhibits 5-lipoxygenase Activity in Leukotriene Synthesis in Rat Basophilic Leukemia-1 Cells," *Journal of Ethnopharmacology,* 48 (1995): 33–41.

17. Y. Tohda, R. Haraguchi, et al., "Effects of Saiboku-to on Dual-phase Bronchoconstriction in Asthmatic Guinea Pigs," *Methods Find Exp Clinical Pharmacology,* 21 (1999): 449–452.

18. Y. Egashira and H. Nagano, "A Multicenter Clinical Trial of TJ-96 in Patients with Steroid-dependent Bronchial Asthma," *Annals of the New York Academy of Sciences,* 685 (1993): 580–583.

19. M. Homma, K. Oka, H. Kobayashi, et al., "Impact of Free Excretions in Asthmatic Patients Who Responded Well to Saiboku-to, a Chinese Herbal Medicine," *Journal of Pharmacy Pharmacology,* 45 (1993): 844–846.

20. S. Nakajima, Y. Tohda, K. Ohkawa, et al., "Effect of Saiboku-to (TJ-96) on Bronchial Asthma," *Annals of the New York Academy of Sciences,* 685 (1993): 549–560.

21. K.V. Thiruvengadam, K. Haranath, S. Sudarsan, et al., "*Tylophora indica* in Bronchial Asthma: A Controlled Comparison with a Standard Anti-asthmatic Drug," *Journal of the Indian Medical Association,* 71 (1978): 172–176.

22. D.N. Shivpuri, M.P.S. Menon, and D. Prakash, "A Cross-over Double-blind Study on *Tylophora indica* in the Treatment of Asthma and Allergic Rhinitis," *Journal of Allergy,* 43 (1969): 145–150.

23. D.N. Shivpuri, S.C. Singhal, and D. Parkash, "Treatment of Asthma with an Alcoholic Extract of *Tylophora indica:* A Crossover, Double-blind Study," *Annals of Allergy,* 30 (1972): 407–412.

Chapter 9: Mind Over Asthma and Other Complementary Therapies

1. B.S. Jonas, D.K. Wagener, J.F. Lando, et al., "Symptoms of Anxiety and Depression as a Risk Factor for the Development of Asthma," *Journal of Applied Biobehavioral Research,* 4 (1999): 91–110.

2. P.J. Brantley and G.N. Jones, "Daily Stress and Stress-related Disorders," *Annals of Behavioral Medicine,* 15 (1993): 17–25. See also: W. Busse, J.K. Kiecolt-Glaser, C. Coe, et al., "Stress and Asthma," *American Journal of Respiratory and Critical Care Medicine,* 151 (1995): 249–252. S. Isenberg, P. Lehrer, and S. Hochron, "The Effects of Suggestion and Emotional Arousal on Pulmonary Function in Asthma: A Review and a Hypothesis Regarding Vagal Medication," *Psychosomatic Medicine,* 54 (1992): 192–216.

3. M.D. Klinnert, E.L. McQuaid, D. McCormick, et al., "A Multimethod Assessment of Behavioral and Emotional Adjustment in Children with Asthma," *Journal of Pediatric Psychology,* 25 (2000): 35–46.

4. S. Gupta, I. Mitchell, R.M. Giuffre, et al., "Covert Fears and Anxiety in Asthma and Congenital Heart Disease," *Child Care Health and Development,* 27 (2001): 335–348.

5. B.D. Miller, and B.L. Wood, "Psychophysiological Reactivity in Asthmatic Children: A Cholinergically Mediated Confluence of Pathways," *Journal of the American Academy of Child and Adolescent Psychiatry,* 33 (1994): 1236–1245.

6. J.M. Smyth, M.H. Soefer, A. Hurewitz, et al., "Daily Psychosocial Factors Predict Levels of Diurnal Cycles of Asthma Symptamatology and Peak Flow," *Journal of Behavioral Medicine,* 22 (1999): 179–193.

7. L.Y. Liu, C.L. Coe, C.A. Swenson, et al., "School Examinations Enhance Airway Inflammation to Antigen Challenge," *American Journal of Respiratory and Critical Care Medicine,* 165 (2002): 1062–1067.

8. C.A. Mancuso, M.G. Peterson, and M.E. Charlson, "Effects of Depressive Symptoms on Health-related Quality of Life in Asthma Patients," *Journal of General Internal Medicine,* 15 (2000): 301–310.

9. S. Centanni, F. Di Marco, F. Castagna, et al., "Psychological Issues in the Treatment of Asthmatic Patients," *Respiratory Medicine,* 94 (2000): 742–749.

10. B.D. Miller and B.L. Wood, "Psychophysiological Reactivity in Asthmatic Children: A Cholinergically Mediated Confluence of Pathways." *Journal of the American Academy of Child and Adolescent Psychiatry,* 33 (1994): 1236–1245.

11. P.M. Lehrer, "Emotionally Triggered Asthma: A Review of Research, Literature, and Some Hypothesis of Self-regulations Therapies," *Applied Psychophysiological Biofeedback,* 23 (1998): 13–41.

12. A. Smith and K. Nicholson, "Psychosocial Factors, Respiratory Viruses and Exacerbation of Asthma." *Psychoneuroendocrinology,* 26 (2001): 411–420.

13. K.B. Thomas, "General Practice Consultations: Is There Any Point in Being Positive?" *British Medical Journal of Clinical Research and Education,* 294 (1987): 1200–1202.

14. P.A. Christensen, L.C. Laursen, E. Taudorf, et al., "Acupuncture and Bronchial Asthma," *Allergy,* 39 (1984): 379–385.

15. K. Linde, K. Jobst, and J. Panton, "Acupuncture for Chronic Asthma," *Cochrane Database Systematic Review,* Issue 1 (2002).

16. C.L. Kern-Buell, A.V. McGrady, P.B. Conran, et al., "Asthma Severity, Psychophysiological Indicators of Arousal, and Immune Function in Asthma Patients Undergoing Biofeedback-assisted Relaxation," *Applied Psychophysiological Biofeedback,* 25 (2000): 79–91.

17. E. Peper and V. Tibbetts, "Fifteen-month Follow-up with Asthmatics Utilizing EMG/Incentive Inspirometer Feedback," *Biofeedback and Self-Regulation,* 17 (1992): 143–151.

18. Available on the Internet: www-camra.ucdavis.edu/RELAXUP.html.

19. H. Kotses, A. Harver, J. Segreto, et al., "Long-term Effects of Biofeedback-induced Facial Relaxation on Measures of Asthma Severity in Children," *Biofeedback and Self-Regulation,* 16 (1991): 1–21.

20. A. McGrady, P. Conran, D. Dickey, et al., "The Effects of Biofeedback-assisted Relaxation on Cell-mediated Immunity, Cortisol, and White Blood Cell Count in Healthy Adult Subjects," *Journal of Behavioral Medicine,* 15 (1992): 343–354.

21. P.M. Lehrer, S.M. Hochron, T. Mayne, et al., "Relationship Between Changes in EMG and Respiratory Sinus Arrhythmia in a Study of Relaxation Therapy for Asthma," *Applied Psychophysiology and Biofeedback,* 22 (1997): 183–191.

22. M. Thomas, R.K. McKinley, E. Freeman, et al., "Prevalence of Dysfunctional Breathing in Patients Treated for Asthma in Primary Care: A Cross-sectional Survey," *British Medical Journal,* 322 (2001): 1098–1100.

23. S.D. Bowler, A. Green, and C.A. Mitchell, "Buteyko Breathing Techniques in Asthma: A Blinded Randomized Controlled Trial," *Medical Journal of Australia,* 169 (1998): 575–578.

24. A.J. Opat, M.M. Cohen, M.J. Bailey, et al., "A Clinical Trial of the Buteyko Breathing Technique in Asthma as Taught by Video," *Journal of Asthma,* 37 (2000): 557–564.

25. G. Bronfort, R.L. Evans, P. Kubic, et al., "Chronic Pediatric Asthma and Chiropractic Spinal Manipulation: A Prospective Clinical Series and Randomized Clinical Pilot Study," *Journal of Manipulative Physiologic Therapy,* 24 (2001): 369–377.

26. N.H. Nielsen, G. Bronfort, T. Bendix, et al., "Chronic Asthma and Chiropractic Spinal Manipulation: A Randomized Clinical Trial," *Clinical Experiment Allergy,* 25 (1995): 80–88.

27. P.M. Lehrer, S.M. Hochron, T. Mayne, et al., "Relaxation and Music Therapies for Asthma Among Patients Prestabilized on Asthma Medication," *Journal of Behavioral Medicine,* 17 (1994): 1–24.

28. R. Lucia, "Effects of Playing a Musical Wind Instrument in Asthmatic Teenagers," *Journal of Asthma,* 31 (1994): 375–385.

29. T.B. Gilbert, "Breathing Difficulties in Wind Instrument Players," *Maryland Medical Journal,* 47 (1998): 23–27.

30. R. Nagarathna and H.R. Nagendra, "Yoga for Bronchial Asthma: A Controlled Study," *British Medical Journal* (*Clinical Research Edition*), 291 (1985): 1077–1079.

31. S.C. Jain and B. Talukdar, "Evaluation of Yoga Therapy Programme for Patients of Bronchial Asthma," *Singapore Medical Journal,* 34 (1993): 306–308.

32. R. Manocha, G.B. Marks, P. Kenchington, et al., "Sahaja Yoga in the Management of Moderate to Severe Asthma: A Randomized Controlled Trial," *Thorax,* 57 (2002): 110–115.

33. J. Panton and E.A. Barley, "Family Therapy for Asthma in Children," *Cochrane Database Systemic Review,* 2 (2000): CD0089.

34. C. Stout, H. Kotses, and T.L. Creer, "Improving Perception of Air Flow Obstruction in Asthma Patients," *Psychosomatic Medicine,* 59 (1997): 201–206.

35. B. Petruson and K. Theman, "Reduced Nocturnal Asthma by Improved Nasal Breathing," *Acta Otolaryngology,* 116 (1996): 490–492.

36. N.M. Ryan-Wenger and M. Walsh, "Children's Perspectives on Coping with Asthma," *Pediatric Nursing,* 20 (1994): 224–228.

Index

A

B

C

D

E

G

H

I

Q

R

S

T

U

V